Daniel Fu Keung Wong, PhD

Clinical Case Management for People with Mental Illness
A Biopsychosocial Vulnerability-Stress Model

Pre-publication
REVIEWS,
COMMENTARIES,
EVALUATIONS . . .

The Haworth Press®
New York • London • Oxford

Clinical Case Management for People with Mental Illness
A Biopsychosocial Vulnerability-Stress Model

HAWORTH *Social Work in Health Care*
Gary Rosenberg and Andrew Wiessman
Editors

Clinical Case Management for People with Mental Illness
A Biopsychosocial Vulnerability-Stress Model

Daniel Fu Keung Wong, PhD

The Haworth Press®
New York • London • Oxford

KH

For more information on this book or to order, visit
http://www.haworthpress.com/store/product.asp?sku=5548

or call 1-800-HAWORTH (800-429-6784) in the United States and Canada
or (607) 722-5857 outside the United States and Canada

or contact orders@HaworthPress.com

The Haworth Press, Inc., 10 Alice Street, Binghamton, NY 13904-1580.

PUBLISHER'S NOTE
The development, preparation, and publication of this work has been undertaken with great care. However, the Publisher, employees, editors, and agents of The Haworth Press are not responsible for any errors contained herein or for consequences that may ensue from use of materials or information contained in this work. The Haworth Press is committed to the dissemination of ideas and information according to the highest standards of intellectual freedom and the free exchange of ideas. Statements made and opinions expressed in this publication do not necessarily reflect the views of the Publisher, Directors, management, or staff of The Haworth Press, Inc., or an endorsement by them.

Identities and circumstances of individuals discussed in this book have been changed to protect confidentiality.

Cover design by Kerry E. Mack.

Library of Congress Cataloging-in-Publication Data

Wong, Daniel Fu Keung.
    Clinical case management for people with mental illness : a biopsychosocial vulnerability-stress model / Daniel Fu Keung Wong.
        p. cm.
    Includes bibliographical references and index.
    ISBN-13: 978-0-7890-2854-9 (hc. : alk. paper)
    ISBN-10: 0-7890-2854-9 (hc. : alk. paper)
    ISBN-13: 978-0-7890-2855-6 (pbk. : alk. paper)
    ISBN-10: 0-7890-2855-7 (pbk. : alk. paper)
    1. Psychiatric social work. 2. Mental health services. 3. Mentally ill—Services for. I. Title.
    [DNLM: 1. Social Work, Psychiatric—methods—Case Reports. 2. Case Management—Case Reports. 3. Community Mental Health Services—Case Reports. 4. Mental Disorders—diagnosis—Case Reports. 5. Mental Disorders—therapy—Case Reports. WM 30.5 W872c 2006]
    HV689.W65 2006
    362.2'0425—dc22
                                                                                            2005012481

6/23/06

CONTENTS

ABOUT THE AUTHOR

Daniel Fu Keung Wong, PhD, is an associate professor of the Department of Social Work and Social Administration at the University of Hong Kong. He is a qualified cognitive therapist who received his training from the Beck Institute in Philadelphia, Pennsylvania. Dr. Wong has worked as a mental health worker in Hong Kong, and as a case manager in Melbourne, Australia.

Foreword

The past two decades have seen marked improvements in the provision of mental health services in Hong Kong with the development of community-based rehabilitation facilities, psychiatric wards attached to district general hospitals, and a younger generation of mental health professionals willing to explore new ways of helping their clients. Numerous articles have been published (in English) in the international and local literature about mental health issues in Hong Kong, but when it comes to a textbook suitable for a local audience that presents a coherent theoretical and practical framework for intervention, a gap exists. This volume fills that gap by providing a clear and accessible model of psychosocial practice with mentally ill people and their families.

An experienced clinician who has worked extensively in both Australia and Hong Kong, Dr. Wong draws on his own practice to provide illuminating insights into useful interventions based on cognitive therapy. He seamlessly integrates theory that was largely developed in Western countries with practice that take place in a Chinese context. The appendixes contain worksheets and checklists that will be of great practical assistance to beginning practitioners. Of particular relevance to social workers is the emphasis that Dr. Wong places on the needs of family members for care as well as on the ways family members can maximize their provision of effective care. This book makes a significant contribution to the Hong Kong literature, and can be warmly recommended to social work teachers and their students as well as to trainees and young practitioners in other relevant professions such as psychiatric nursing and occupational therapy.

Veronica Pearson, PhD
Department of Social Work
and Social Administration
The University of Hong Kong

Preface

This book introduces a clinical case management approach for assessing and working with people suffering from depression, anxiety disorders, schizophrenia, and personality disorders; for helping family members cope; and for handling psychiatric emergencies. Theoretically, a biopsychosocial vulnerability-stress model is used for understanding the dynamic interplay among the biological, psychological, social, and environmental factors that influence the course of development and the severity of a person's mental illness.

It is argued that successful clinical case management relies on a clear understanding of the relationships between the aforementioned factors and the creative use of different therapeutic approaches in helping an individual suffering from mental disorder. The book describes this model clearly, using clinical experiences in Hong Kong and Australia as examples to illustrate various points. Each chapter contains at least one detailed case example that thoroughly delineates the assessment and intervention processes of clinical case management. Chapter 1 introduces the concepts and contexts of clinical case management, and Chapters 2 and 3 provide a detailed description of the biopsychosocial stress-vulnerability model and its application in conducting a thorough psychiatric assessment. Chapters 4 through 7 present ways in which this model can be used to manage an individual suffering from depression, anxiety disorder, schizophrenia, or personality disorder. Chapter 8 focuses on helping family members with relatives suffering from mental illnesses. Finally, Chapter 9 provides readers with the knowledge and skills for handling suicide and psychiatric violence.

This book is particularly written for mental health professionals in such fields as social work, psychiatric nursing, and occupational therapy. It not only provides frameworks for assessment and intervention for working with people suffering from major mental disorders, it also introduces readers to practical intervention skills that are based on the author's own clinical experiences. Plenty of case examples are offered to help readers understand the concepts and theories relating to the different frameworks of assessment and intervention, and worksheets are included that illustrate the clinical skills used in the assessment and intervention processes.

Chapter 1

Clinical Case Management:
An Overview

INTRODUCTION

Mental health workers function within certain political, social, and economic contexts in a society. This chapter introduces these contexts by giving an account of the development of mental health services in Hong Kong, a critique of the mental health services, and an explanation of the difficulties faced by mental health workers when delivering services to their clients in Hong Kong. The second part of this chapter is devoted to discussing the concept of clinical case management and how this concept has been developed to work with two broadly differentiated groups of people with mental illness: individuals with mild mental illness and individuals with chronic mental illness. Differences exist in the nature and skills of clinical case management for people suffering from mild mental illness and those suffering from chronic mental illness. Generally speaking, whereas the emphasis for working with people with chronic mental illness (e.g., schizophrenia) centers on rehabilitation and supportive counseling, the focus of intervention for people suffering from mild mental illness (e.g., anxiety disorders) revolves around cure and in-depth, therapeutic counseling.

MENTAL HEALTH SERVICES IN HONG KONG:
A CRITICAL REVIEW

Development of Community-Based Mental Health Services in Hong Kong

At least three driving forces led to the development of community care in Hong Kong. These forces were quite similar to those found in other developed countries, and included: (1) adverse effects of institutionalization, (2) advent of psychotropic medications, and (3) benefits of community living.

Adverse Effects of Institutionalization

The effects of institutionalization were strongly criticized in the 1960s and 1970s. In a classic movie, *One Flew Over the Cuckoo's Nest* (1975), patients had to conform to strict rules and regulations in an oppressive psychiatric hospital. In the movie, patients were confined to a locked-up environment without any programs for rehabilitation. Some patients escaped into their illnesses in order to survive the institutional oppression. Others were apathetic and showed no interest in their living environment. The movie was said to reflect a certain reality of psychiatric hospitals at the time, and understandably, this and many other incidents aroused the public attention toward improving the lives of people with mental illness. Consequently, a movement toward deinstitutionalization of mental patients began.

Advent of Psychotropic Medications

It would not be possible for some chronically mentally ill patients with severe psychotic symptoms to live in the community without the support of psychotropic medications. Indeed, these medications were, and still are, able to help control clients' symptoms. With the intake of medications, many chronically ill patients are able to function adequately in the community. The earliest publicly used psychotropic medication was chlorpromazine (Torrey, 1988). Therefore, the advent of psychotropic medications could be seen as a positive driving force toward deinstitutionalization and community care for people with chronic mental illness.

Benefits of Community Living

Since the 1960s, some countries, such as the United States and Great Britain, have begun to experiment with different types of community-based mental health programs for persons with mental illness. These programs have been introduced with the understanding that in-vivo training in community living is a better treatment modality for persons with mental illness than hospital care (Test & Stein, 2000). Moreover, it may foster a sense of community spirit among citizens. Thus, community-based mental health programs such as assertive outreach, psychiatric crisis assessment and treatment team, halfway houses, small group homes, and sheltered employment have been established (Test & Stein, 2000). Many of these programs underwent evaluations and were found to bring beneficial effects such as reduced hospital stay, fewer hospitalizations, better social functioning, and better quality of life for persons with chronic mental illness (Test & Stein, 2000). In Hong Kong, studies have been carried out to examine the effectiveness of some currently run community mental health services, such as the community psychiatric team services (Chiu, Poon, Fong, & Tsoh, 2000) and long-term care homes (Cheung, 2001). However, no comprehensive review or policy evaluation of mental health services has yet been done in Hong Kong.

Time Line of Development of Mental Health Services in Hong Kong

The Early Days: Custodial Care

Prior to World War II, no community-based psychiatric service was available for people with mental illness in Hong Kong. These individuals were put into asylums run by charitable organizations, such as Tung Wah services. Some of them might also be sent to Fong Chuen Hospital in Guangzhou, China. Services were custodial in nature and the Hong Kong government did not take an active role in financing and providing services for people with mental illness (Yip, 1998).

The 1960s and 1970s: The Introduction of an Infrastructure of Mental Health Services

The establishment of the infrastructure of inpatient and outpatient mental health services began after World War II (Yip, 1998). The Castle Peak Hospital, one of the largest psychiatric hospitals in Hong Kong, was opened in 1961. Community-based facilities, such as halfway houses and sheltered workshops for mentally ill persons, were also established during this period. In addition, the Mental Health Ordinance was enacted at around the same time as well. However, although hospital-based psychiatric services were still largely custodial in nature, community-based psychiatric rehabilitation services were far and few (Yip, 1998). For example, very few halfway house placements were available for persons with mental illness before 1982. Moreover, these houses were managed on a twenty-four-hour basis, seven days a week, by one social work diploma holder and two nontrained welfare workers. In the case of vocational rehabilitation services, with the exception of a few sheltered workshops, little vocational training and employment-assisted programs, such as supported employment and day training centers for persons with mental illness, were available. Indeed, community-based psychiatric rehabilitation services did not take shape until the early 1980s. During these early days of the development of mental health services, the basic skeleton of medical, social, and vocational rehabilitation services had begun to form. However, the movement to deinstitutionalize mentally ill persons had not been fully recognized by the government.

The Consolidation of Mental Health Services

In 1982, an acutely psychotic person went into a kindergarten in Kowloon, Hong Kong, killing and injuring a number of children. This incident created a scare in the community. As a consequence, the government formed a task force and subsequently made several recommendations for improving community-based psychiatric services in Hong Kong. For example, community psychiatric nursing services were introduced and halfway houses for persons with mental illness were greatly expanded, with a new staffing structure that included social workers, psychiatric nurses, welfare workers, and minor staff. Other services, such as day training centers, aftercare services, longstay care homes, and carer support groups, were gradually introduced to the community psychiatric rehabilitation service structure in Hong Kong. To further protect the interest of the public as well as the right of persons with mental illness, the Mental Health Ordinance was also revised. During this period the government took more responsibility in financing social and vocational rehabilitation services in Hong Kong. However, residential services were still institutional in nature, with each halfway house and long-stay care home taking forty and two hundred residents respectively. Yet, with the rapid expansion of community-based psychiatric services in Hong Kong, psychiatric stigma surfaced as an important issue of grave concern (Hong Kong Council of Social Services & MHAHK, 1996). The public was found to hold very negative and even hostile attitudes toward persons with mental illness. Indeed, many community psychiatric services had to be built in remote areas or with front entrances put in locations that were not easily accessible to the public.

It was during this period that the call for the establishment of a case management system was raised among professionals in the mental health field. This included a number of issues. First, with the rapid and extensive expansion of community-based rehabilitation services, the lack of coordination between the inpatient hospital services and the community-based psychiatric services, and between different types of community-based services was criticized. Complaints about the delay in accessing services, the rigid criteria for admission to services, and the inadequate services in the community were heard. Second, since clients may receive a multitude of services from different mental health professionals, it would be sensible to identify a key worker who would oversee the coordination of services for the clients. However, mental health workers, family members, and clients had difficulty choosing the key workers. It was not clear to them who should be responsible for coordinating services for the clients. A system to designate the key person accountable to the welfare of the client needed to be created. Third, since many clients were rather chronic and passive, the clients had difficulty asserting their rights and negotiating their needs with the health care professionals in the mental health system. Professionals were needed to help these individuals advocate their rights. In spite of these needs, the government has not yet formally adopted a case management approach as part of the mental health care system, even to this date. In contrast, in the United States, case management has been included as one of the key components in the service delivery system in mental health care (Levine & Fleming, 1984).

The 1990s to Present: The Experimentations of New Mental Health Services

Since the establishment of the Hospital Authority (HA) in Hong Kong in the early 1990s, psychiatric inpatient and community rehabilitation services have undergone many changes. A number of specialized, community-based psychiatric services have been established. These include such initiatives as community psychiatric treatment (CPT) teams for crisis assessment and management services, psychogeriatric assessment and treatment services, and early assessment service for young people with psychosis (EASY). Indeed, under the governance of HA in Hong Kong, a trend toward developing inpatients and community-based specialized psychiatric services (e.g., for the elderly, youth, and children with special needs) has begun. Mental health professionals have begun to experiment with new medical and psychosocial intervention approaches in helping their clients. For example, different intervention programs and psychotherapies, such as cognitive therapists and social skills training, have been used to help people with different mental health problems.

Under the Social Welfare Department (SWD), attempts have also been made to shorten the waiting list for different types of community-based rehabilitation services by building more halfway houses and long-stay care homes. In vocational rehabilitation, supported employment as a new initiative was launched in the mid-1990s. A new service called mental health link was also introduced in the mental health care system in early 2000.

Issues and Problems of Mental Health Services in Hong Kong

Several issues and problems confront the mental health care system in Hong Kong. These are explained in the following sections.

Lack of Direction and Coordination of Service

In Hong Kong, the Health, Welfare and Foods Bureau is designated to be in charge of the overall coordination of health care related services, including mental health services. Three parties are involved in the provision of mental health services in Hong Kong: The HA, SWD, and the Department of Health. The HA provides inpatient and medically related community-based rehabilitation services, and the SWD renders mainly community-based social, residential, and vocational rehabilitation services to persons with mental illness. The Department of Health provides prevention services such as public education for the general population (Health and Welfare Bureau, 1999).

Under this structure, several questions may be raised. On the policy level, although it is encouraging to find that various parties have deployed resources to develop different mental health programs, no clear, overall policy direction guides the development of mental health services in Hong Kong. For example, what is the best mix for hospital and community-based rehabilitation services in Hong Kong? In some parts of the world, resources resulting from the closure of psychiatric hospitals have been devoted to developing community-based psychiatric rehabilitation services (Australian Health Ministers, 1992). In Hong Kong, a larger proportion of the health care resources for psychiatric services are still put into supporting hospital services (Health and Welfare Bureau, 1999). Whereas various political, social, and cultural conditions may have shaped the development and setting of different priorities in different countries, the Hong Kong SAR (Special Administrative Region) government still has not established an overall mental health policy to guide the development of mental health services in Hong Kong, even though various mental health acts have been legally endorsed in such countries as the United States, the United Kingdom, and Canada.

Other important questions that need to be asked are What is the best possible model of community rehabilitation services for Hong Kong? and What specific types of community-based services should be further developed? Lawson (1995), invited by the government to examine the mental health services in Hong Kong, proposed a cluster-based model of mental health service. According to the model, each cluster consists of psychiatric beds located in general hospitals, an outpatient clinic, a CPT team, vocational rehabilitation services, and residential services. This type of cluster-based service model has been successful in other countries. Unfortunately, his idea had not been fully adopted by the Hong Kong government.

On the practice level, mental health professionals from the HA and the SWD have complained about the delay in service provision due to rigid admission procedures and criteria (Yip, 1997). For example, some hospital staff commented about the long delay in processing and formally admitting a client into halfway houses. Other staff found that the CPT teams are unable to respond quickly to their request for assisting clients in crisis. Central to these complaints is a difference in judgment among different service personnel regarding the severity and urgency of the conditions and the needs of clients.

Confusion exists as well regarding the admission criteria set by different units offering similar services. For example, staff commented that different CPT teams have different sets of service criteria. Some teams manage only cases that were discharged from their own hospitals and do not reach out and assess potential outside cases. Another example is complaints that the staff of some halfway houses interpret their admission criteria more stringently than others, thus refusing to admit certain clients who would otherwise be accepted in a different house.

Inadequate Delivery of Mental Health Services

Experiences in the United States and Britain have suggested that assertive outreach is an essential characteristic of a good community support system for persons with mental illness, particularly those with chronic mental illness. Services should also be continuous with no definite time frame. In Hong Kong, except for community psychiatric nurses (CPNs) and CPT teams, the dominant service delivery mode is still largely office-based ,with a nine-to-five working schedule. Very few services operate on the weekends and after office hours. Clients with chronic mental illness who are passive and/or resistant to treatment may not be able to receive timely interventions when needed. Indeed, evidence has shown that delays in seeking psychiatric treatment are a common and serious issue needing the attention of the mental health professionals (Chiu et al., 2000). Mental health services that bear an assertive outreach component and operate after office hours may be able to address the issues of the delay in treatment and prevent hospitalization.

Continuous support, particularly by an identifiable person in a trusting relationship, is crucial for persons with chronic mental illness. Current practices of mental health services such as medical social services and halfway houses have a definite time frame, and no single, identifiable person assists the client throughout his or her rehabilitation process. This service delivery mode may not serve the best interest of clients with chronic mental illness because these individuals need mental health professionals who have a working knowledge of their mental health conditions, patterns of relapse, coping skills, and support systems; with whom they have developed a trusting relationship; and who can provide continuous support for them.

Moreover, whereas some clients with chronic mental illness require continuous support from mental health workers, others may need assistance from mental health workers only at certain period of time during the course of their rehabilitation. Continuity is certainly needed.

Lack of Community Rehabilitation Services

According to the Hong King *Rehabilitation Programme Plan Review* (Health and Welfare Bureau, 1999), shortfalls exist in services such as halfway houses and long-stay care homes. For example, the shortfalls in estimated demand for residental placements in long-stay care homes and halfway house placements for the year of 2002-2003 were 1,643 and 948, respectively. Available parent/relatives resource centers are also lacking. Currently, four government subsidized resource centers are available, but three of these four centers have been funded by the SWD only since October 2003. In addition, some mentally ill clients who work full time have expressed their need for extended hours of psychiatric consultation, particularly in the evenings and weekends.

Lack of Use of Informal Care

Advocates of the use of informal care maintain that mental health professionals are not fully aware of the needs and problems of persons with mental illness (Hatfield & Lefley, 1987). They claim that relatives know more clearly the needs and problems of the person with the illness than do the professionals. A study conducted by Spaniol, Jung, Zipple, & Fitzgerald (1987) found that family members and clients themselves had significantly lower levels of satisfaction toward various mental health services than those of the mental health professionals. They suggested the establishment of self-help or mutual-aid organizations to help family members. Indeed, overseas experiences have shown that these self-help organizations play a pivotal role in shaping the development of mental health services (Torrey, 1988). These organizations provide psychoeducation, mutual support, and advocacy for persons with chronic mental illness and their family members. In Hong Kong, as previosly mentioned, only four government-subsidized parents/relatives resource centers exist along with a few self-help groups with small memberships. The mental health care system has not fully utilized the resources available from these informal and networks.

Lack of Resources for Persons Suffering from Mild Symptoms of Psychiatric Illness

At present, most of the resources in mental health care have been put into services for persons with serious mental illness, such as schizophrenia, and very few resources have been devoted to establishing services for individuals suffering from mild symptoms of psychiatric illness, such as anxiety disorders and depression (Health and Welfare Bureau, 1999). According to Hong Kong government statistics, many individuals with chronic mental illness utilize rehabilitation services, and only about 1.5 percent of individuals with mild psychiatric illness utilize rehabilitation services. The Hong Kong government has adamantly maintained that persons with mild mental illness can obtain services from existing medical social services and family services. In reality, some of these service units do not have the manpower or time to provide in-depth individual and group counseling for these individuals. Furthermore, some workers may not have the clinical knowledge and skills in mental health to perform psychiatric assessment and counseling for persons with such illnesses. With an increase in the number of persons with mild psychiatric illness in Hong Kong, the government needs to administer more resources to agencies that provide individual and group counseling for people suffering from mild psychiatric illness such as anxiety disorders.

Stigmatization of Mental Illness

As previously mentioned, psychiatric stigma has seriously affected the development of mental health services in Hong Kong. Two studies conducted by the joint effort of Hong Kong Council of Social Services and The Mental Health Association of Hong Kong (MHAHK) (1996, 1997) suggest that the majority of 1,043 respondents were quite negative about mental patients and mental health facilities. This negative attitude has direct impacts on the lives of persons with mental illness. They are socially disadvantaged. One study conducted by Pearson et al. (2003) found that persons who had a label of mental illness were less likely to be granted a job interview than were other disabled groups. Psychiatric stigma may extend to a person's daily life, particularly for those with overt residual symptoms. They may be ridiculed by passersby, colleagues, and even family members. This may lead to adverse personal reactions such as low self-esteem.

ROLES AND FUNCTIONS
OF MENTAL HEALTH WORKERS:
A CLINICAL CASE MANAGEMENT PERSPECTIVE

Concept of Clinical Case Management

Case management is conceived as one of the ten essential components of a community support system for persons with mental illness (Levine & Fleming, 1984). While it aims to redress some of the inherent problems and issues of mental health service systems, it also attempts to serve rehabilitative and therapeutic functions. Psychiatric rehabilitation services are diverse and often involve different governmental departments (e.g., the SWD and HA) and different professionals (e.g., nurses, psychologists, psychiatrists, and social workers). It is not uncommon to hear comments about problems in the system, such as fragmentation of services, lack of accountability, and unnecessary delay in receiving the appropriate services (Yip, 1997). Case management coordinates these services and the service providers involved and helps the individuals with mental illness to access these services as smoothly and as timely as possible. Indeed, case management ensures continuity of care for persons with mental illness. Moreover, under case management, each client is assigned a case manager. This individual case manager assists the client in negotiating the different systems so that he or she may receive the necessary and appropriate care. The case manager must ensure that all service providers, including himself or herself, are accountable for the welfare of the clients. In sum, case management aims to ensure continuity of services, client's accessibility to services, service providers' accountability to the welfare of the client, and timely services for clients.

Besides solving some of the inherent problems in the mental health service system, case management also provides important therapeutic and rehabilitative services. A case manager is a therapeutic agent who not only performs the linkage work but also provides the support and counseling necessary for client's personal growth. Walsh (2000) argues that case management is therapeutic and that it incorporates the essence of psychotherapy. His argument stems from the process of interaction between a case manager and a client for the purpose of improving the client's disability or malfunction regarding cognitive, affective, and/or behavioral functions. Specifically, a case manager performs the following therapeutic functions: identifying early signs of relapse and unmanageable stress; assessing environmental impacts on client's functioning; motivating the client to participate in treatment; helping the client manage his or her cognitive, affective, and/or behavioral malfunctions; and developing the client's inner potential (Walsh, 2000). In general, a case manager provides: (1) assessment, (2) service planning, (3) linkage, (4) advocacy, (5) counseling therapy, (6) monitoring of services, and (7) evaluation (Rapp, 1998a).

Assessment

Broadly speaking, assessment is of the needs, strengths, and limitations of a client. Specifically, assessment focuses on such issues as the impact of psychiatric impairments on the functioning of the individual, the societal constraints that affect the client's access to resources, and the client's psychological reactions toward his or her illness. Indeed, a case manager needs to have adequate understanding of the dynamic interplay of the different personal, social, and environmental forces that affect the rehabilitation process of a person with mental illness. In order to do so, a case manager must have some knowledge about the medical aspects of mental illness as well as the social and psychological theories related to mental illness. (This is discussed in further detail in Chapter 2.)

Service Planning

After careful assessment, the case manager must provide a treatment plan for his or her client. In the plan, the case manager should choose the types of services and treatment that will best address the identified problems, potentials, and limitations of the client. He or she must identify where, when, and how the client will receive these services and treatment. In this regard, the case manager must be aware of the most current resources available in the mental health care system, the boundaries of various types of services, and the procedures in obtaining these services.

Linkage

Linkage may seem simple, and literally means linking the client to appropriate services, but in reality it is a rather difficult step in the case management process. Among the available services, the case manager must know the working cultures of the related service agencies and styles of the workers involved. He or she must learn the skills needed to negotiate with workers of these agencies and must be able to safeguard the welfare of the client.

Advocacy

Advocacy work is performed on two levels: individual and systems. On the individual level, the case manager attempts to redress any injustice that is done to the client as soon as he or she is aware of it (e.g., a mental health worker intervenes after hearing that an employer deliberately reduced his or her client's salary because of the client's mental illness). On the systems level, a case manager attempts to change the policies, procedures, and practices that create injustice for or inhibits the rights of persons with mental illness (e.g., mental health workers have been advocating the establishment of nighttime clinics for clients who cannot attend clinics during the day).

Counseling and Therapy

A case manager offers supportive counseling, guiding the client at every step of his or her rehabilitation process. Activities may include emotional support, advice and assistance, and even social companionship. A case manager with advanced training in counseling and therapy can help an individual client improve his or her cognitive, affective, and/or behavioral functioning, and can help enhance his or her potential and personal growth as well. This book is devoted to helping readers acquire knowledge and develop the initial competence needed to be a clinical case manager.

Monitoring of Services

Service monitoring requires the case manager to "keep an eye" on the services to ensure that they continuously meet the needs of the client. In fact, the case manager must be sensitive to the changing needs of the client, and must make necessary adjustments to the treatment plan and programs.

Evaluation

The two levels of evaluation in case management are evaluation of the process and of the outcome. The case manager must evaluate the program's effectiveness based on whether his or her therapeutic inputs during the process have made an impact on the client's rehabilitation outcome. Both the process (e.g., therapeutic inputs) and the outcome (e.g., efficiency and effectiveness) should be evaluated. The evaluation should be ongoing throughout the rehabilitation process. This is very important, because as the client's needs and circumstances change, services and treatment may have to be adjusted to meet his or her changing needs. Therefore, the case manager needs to engage the client in ongoing assessment, planning, monitoring, and evaluation of situations, services, and treatments.

Models of Case Management

A variety of models of case management are practiced (Levine & Fleming, 1984). These may be conveniently labeled as (1) a generalist/rehabilitation model, (2) a clinical model, or (3) a volunteer case management model. These models differ in terms of the types of case management functions they emphasize and the types of personnel carrying out the case management activities. However, in actual practice, it is difficult to identify any pure model that fits the following exact descriptions.

Generalist/Rehabilitation Model

A case manager performs assessment, service planning, linkage, advocacy, supportive counseling, monitoring of the client's rehabilitation process, and evaluation. Under the umbrella of this generalist/rehabilitation model, the case manager is expected to perform a great deal of linkage and support functions. He or she draws on the diverse community-based rehabilitation services available and works closely with other professionals in helping clients with mental illness. Meanwhile, the case manager continues to provide instrumental and emotional support for the client throughout the rehabilitation process. Case managers must have some college education, particularly in the social sciences, and will also need ongoing training to help them carry out the various case management activities. Currently, this model is widely adopted in many countries. The PACT (programs of assertive community treatment) or ACT (assertive community treatment) programs in the United States of America (e.g., Santos et al., 1993) and aftercare services in Hong Kong bear much resemblance to this generalist/rehabilitation model.

Clinical Model

In the clinical model, a case manager performs similar functions to those described in the generalist/rehabilitation model. However, he or she is expected to render counseling and therapy for individuals with mental illness. The case manager in the case must have additional and advanced training in counseling and psychotherapy. This model is particularly suitable for high-risk mentally ill clients or for those needing in-depth counseling. Some teams using this model adopt a specialist stance, and team members may include psychiatrists, psychologists, social workers, nurses, and occupational therapists. In Hong Kong, some of the EASY teams (for individuals with early psychosis) can be seen as partially adopting this clinical case management model.

Volunteer Case Management Model

The case manager is a volunteer who helps a client with chronic mental illness perform day-to-day activities, usually on a one-to-one basis. The case manager may accompany the client to medical follow-ups, shopping, social and recreational activities, etc. An agency staff provides regular supervision for the volunteer case manager. The driving force for running this type of program is to foster the atmosphere of a caring community. The Welcome Basket project run in the United States is an example of how to accomplish this (e.g., Chinman, Weingarten, Stayner, & Davidson, 2001).

Clinical Case Management In Hong Kong:
Potential and Limitations

As mentioned earlier, adopting a case management approach as part of the overall mental health care system offers many advantages. Such a system may address some of the problems evident in the mental health care system in Hong Kong. In clinical case management, a case manager is able to coordinate and negotiate with different departments and different professionals, thus reducing the potential barriers arising from conflicting professional views on the client's needs on rigid admission criteria for different service units. Consequently, this may ensure smoother access to services. Moreover, a case manager is active in reaching out to the clients, particularly to those who are passive and withdrawn. The setting up of a case management system may be particularly useful for persons with very serious mental illness for whom discharge from hospitals and long-term care facilities would be unlikely (Intagliata, 1982).

Although obvious advantages are evident for setting up a case management system in Hong Kong, the Hong Kong government has not fully initiated this in the mental health care system. One reason for the lack of enthusiasm may be because the current structure of mental health care system would have to undergo some reorganization in order for clinical case management to happen. Collaboration and reallocation of resources among different departments such as the SWD and the HA would be needed, and staff of these units would have to be trained in case management and community psychiatry. What is most difficult to achieve, perhaps, is the rethinking needed to and develop a model for community-based psychiatric services that is agreeable to all parties concerned. It may be more feasible to first explore the possibility of adopting partial case management for specific target population of mentally ill persons in Hong Kong. At present, a few mental health programs, such as aftercare service projects for people discharged from halfway houses and the EASY teams for young people with psychosis in Hong Kong, appear to have adopted a case management model. These programs can serve as prototypes for other target groups in Hong Kong, such as the chronically mentally ill and elderly suffering from dementia.

Target Population for Clinical Case Management

According to the *Rehabilitation Programme Plan Review* (Health and Welfare Bureau, 1999), a total of about 960,000 people in Hong Kong suffer from various kinds of mental illness. As mentioned, mental illness can be conveniently divided into two major categories: chronic and mild. It is important to distinguish these two major categories because the conceptualization of problems and the focus of case management activities differ between these two groups.

Chronic Mental Illness

Defining chronic mental illness. Schizophrenia, manic depression, depression, organic brain-related issues, and similar diseases may be classified as chronic mental illness. According to *Diagnostic and Statistical Manual of Mental Disorders* (DSM-IV-TR) (American Psychiatric Association, 2000), these illnesses constitute conditions that seriously affect the social and occupational functioning and/or personality of an individual. For example, some clients with a chronic condition cannot even perform such simple and basic self-care activities as brushing their teeth. A number of factors may account for the severe loss in functioning, one of which is related to the occurrence of residual symptoms. Symptoms may take the forms of positive or negative symptoms. For example, one of my clients often experienced visual hallucination when he was under stress, and complained about "seeing a cross turning in his head." This hallucination constantly induced distress in him, and consequently he had to take leave and return to the halfway house for rest. Negative symptoms may be poor concentration, lack of motivation, and flattened affect. From my clinical experiences, many residents of halfway houses and long-term care homes in Hong Kong exhibit a great number of negative symptoms. These clients appear passive and do not have much energy to engage in daily and social activities and are often difficult to motivate.

Psychological factors may also play a part in creating a severe loss of functioning among persons with mental illness. Some individuals experience such psychological issues as a lack of acceptance of illness, a sense of loss associated with being unable to perform in the same way as he or she once could, and shame and guilt of being a mentally ill person, particularly in a society with strong psychiatric stigma such as Hong Kong. These issues can dishearten the individual and produce a sense of hopelessness. Consequently, the individual with a mental illness may withdraw from social participation, leading to poor social and occupational functioning.

Two issues are closely related to the chronicity of mental illness. Regarding the duration of mental illness, for some clients the illness can be lifelong. The course of illness is not a linear process. Some individuals experience periods of relative stability and intermittent relapses. They usually require continuous medications and medical follow-ups. As a general rule, the more relapses an individual has, the poorer his or her prognosis. Another issue regarding chronicity is repeated hospitalizations. At present, people with serious mental illness need to take medications continuously, and a close relationship exists between noncompliance to medications and psychiatric relapses (Mueser & Gingerich, 1994). People who do not comply with medications have a higher risk of relapse and thus a greater chance of hospitalization. Side effects of medications and a lack of insight about mental illness are two major reasons for noncompliance (this will be discussed in details in Chapter 6). Without medications, many of these individuals have to be hospitalized.

Clinical case management for persons with chronic mental illness. Most clients receiving psychiatric rehabilitation services in Hong Kong are persons with chronic mental illness. According to the *Rehabilitation Programme Plan Review* (Health and Welfare Bureau, 1999), of the estimated 960,000 mentally ill people in Hong Kong, only about 20 percent suffer from serious mental illness. However, they consume more than 70 percent of the psychiatric rehabilitation services. The focus of clinical case management for these individuals is not about cure, but about rehabilitation (Wing & Morris, 1981). Bridges, Huxley, and Oliver (1994) define psychiatric rehabilitation as "a process which aims to minimize the negative effects of the dynamic relationships between biological, psychological, functional and environmental factors, and maximize the person's latent abilities and strengths." The long-term goal is to help a person travel through an illness at minimal personal cost and maximal personal benefit, particularly in terms of achieving an optimal level of functioning and well-being—even if the illness has a deteriorating course. Indeed, clinical case management attempts to help these individuals with chronic mental illness maintain their optimal social and occupational functioning despite their strong and persistent residual symptoms: poor self-care and daily living skills, poor social relationships and networks, high level of dependence, risk of harm to self or others, poor motivation, impaired capacity for self-management, and vocational difficulties.

According to Wing and Morris (1981), a person's level of psychiatric disability varies according to the interplay among three major components: psychiatric impairments, social disadvantages, and personal reactions to illness. A closer examination of these components provides insight into the focus of assessment and interventions relating to clinical case management.

Psychiatric impairments refer to the severity of symptoms experienced by the persons with serious mental illness. Two persons suffering from schizophrenia may have different levels of psychiatric impairments depending on the presence or severity of their positive and negative residual symptoms. Generally speaking, people with severe residual symptoms have greater psychiatric impairments and are often more disabled. One of the focuses of intervention is to minimize the occurrence and impact of these residual symptoms on the persons. Psychotropic medications help control the symptoms, however, psychological and social interventions can also help the individual learn to control and adjust to these symptoms. For example, with clinical case management, a person experiencing auditory hallucinations will probably be given medications, and is likely to be learning cognitive behavioral strategies to manage the hallucinations as well, thus reducing its impact on his or her daily functioning.

Social disadvantages refer to the deprived and hostile environments that aggravate the social and occupational functioning of persons with chronic mental illness. Disadvantages may include psychiatric stigma, poverty, unemployment, and homelessness. According to Wing and Morris (1981), social disadvantages tend to accumulate over the years. In other words, the older one gets, the greater the impact of these social disadvantageous conditions on the persons with serious mental illness. The focus of intervention is to redress these social disadvantage by either helping the individual develop capabilities to overcome the disadvantages or by changing the environmental conditions to be more conducive to the person's rehabilitation process. For example, vocational skills training programs can help the individual to acquire skills and be more competitive in the open job markets, and educational programs can help reduce psychiatric stigma among employers, which may help create more job opportunities for the individual with the illness.

Personal reactions to illness simply refer to how the person appraises his or her illness situation. The more negatively he or she perceives his or her condition to be, the more adverse the person's psychological reactions will be. Indeed, people with chronic mental illness commonly have low self-esteem. It is understandable because, due to psychiatric impairments, some of them cannot function in the same way they did in the past. They also have to deal with the socially disadvantageous illness label they have acquired. As mentioned, one's level of adverse personal reactions to illness is closely related to the severity of his or her psychiatric impairments and social disadvantages. Supportive counseling is often mentioned as a sucessful approach toward working with individuals with a chronic mental illness. (Details of this approach will be discussed in Chapter 6.)

Case example. Ah Lee was an intelligent Form 7 (twelfth grade) secondary school graduate who had developed schizophrenia at the age of twenty-two, and was referred to our halfway house after a two-year stay in the hospital. Ah Lee repeatedly failed the university entrance examination even though his brother was a graduate of a local university in Hong Kong. According to the medical staff of the hospital, when Ah Lee was first hospitalized, he tended to coil up in bed in a fetal position. He refused to get out of bed and was highly inactive. This passivity continued while he was living in the halfway house. He did not seem to have any motivation to do anything. To make matters worse, he had active auditory hallucinations, with a female voice calling him a "good for nothing" person. He claimed he had difficulty concentrating during conversation and had to repeatedly move his arm in circular motion so that he could have energy to talk to others. Generally, he had profound symptoms that seriously affected his participation in his social and vocational rehabilitation programs.

This put him in a rather socially disadvantageous position because he had not been able to develop the adequate social and vocational skills essential for community living. Indeed, upon meeting this young man, one could not help but quickly feel his hopelessness and low self-esteem. During the initial assessment, Ah Lee and I identified several issues that he was facing: (1) severe psychiatric impairments, which included auditory hallucinations, poor concentration, suicidal ideation, lack of volition, and anhedonia; (2) lack of prevocational, vocational, social, and independent living skills; and (3) very low self-esteem and lack of confidence. Along with arranging the necessary community psychiatric services for Ah Lee, I agreed to meet with him weekly. In the interviews, while monitoring his mental state, I also talked with him about his concerns and interests in life. It was in one of these interviews that he told me that he used to enjoy playing badminton and table tennis. With encouragement, he started to play table tennis with another client and a staff member in the halfway house. This turned out to be a major turning point in his rehabilitation process. After a while, he claimed he "regained some energy," and was able to participate a bit more in social and vocational activities.

However slow the process was, we felt that Ah Lee was moving toward the goals of gaining more confidence in himself, participating socially and vocationally, and learning strategies to deal with his auditory hallucinations. This illustration tells us that rehabilitation for persons with chronic conditions is a very slow and gradual process, and requires the support of a multitude of inpatient and community psychiatric rehabilitation services, and, above all, it requires the support of the staff, particularly the case manager. Yet, the ultimate objective is not cure or full recovery for the person, but instead to develop his or her potential. The word *gradual* denotes a very important meaning in psychiatric rehabilitation, as rehabilitation requires careful assessment and planning to develop the person's potential as he or she gains more and more confidence and ability. At times mental health professionals may make a mistake of pushing clients to achieve certain goals for which they are not ready, thus leading to unnecessary stress and distress in the clients.

In the process of Ah Lee's rehabilitation, the worker performed different case management activities. First, the worker conducted a very careful assessment of Ah Lee and examined the severity of his psychiatric impairments, his social disadvantageous conditions, and his adverse personal reactions to his illness. It was apparent that his psychiatric impairments and adverse personal reactions had severely disabled him, making him particularly vulnerable to internal and external stressors. The worker continuously assessed and monitored the mental state of Ah Lee, particularly during his various transitional periods. While the worker helped Ah Lee make realistic rehabilitation plans and referred him to appropriate rehabilitation services in the community, he also provided continuous counseling and support to Ah Lee, preparing him to go through various stressful moments in his rehabilitation process.

Mild Mental Illness

Defining mild mental illness. About 78 percent of people in Hong Kong suffering from a mental illness belong in this category (Health and Welfare Bureau, 1999). People with mild symptoms of psychiatric illness are those who receive medical or psychological treatment in the community. Only very few receive inpatient psychiatric rehabilitation services. Anxiety disorders, depression (depression can also fall into the category of chronic mental illness), and some neurotic disorders are the most common types of mental illnesses that are grouped under the category of mild mental illness. In the *Rehabilitation Programme Plan Review* (Health and Welfare Bureau, 1999), most of these individuals are categorized as people with a "neurosis." Although the number of people suffering from mild mental illness is large, only 16 percent of these individuals are estimated to require rehabilitation services. The majority receive counseling services from private counselors, counseling service centers, family service centers, and/or receive medical treatments from the government and private medical clinics.

Clinical case management for persons with mild mental illness. People suffering from chronic mental illness experience continuous and sometimes deteriorating mental conditions. In contrast, individuals with mild mental illness normally experience only periodic disruptions to some aspects of their social and occupational functioning. Indeed, the impact of mental illness on these individuals is comparatively less severe, and it is quite possible for these individuals to achieve full recovery from their illnesses. For example, a client with depression is able to maintain his or her usual occupation, although he or she may need to have a break from time to time due to recurrent depressive episodes. Moreover, he or she is not likely to experience any major change in personality nor does the illness exert a long-term effect on the social and occupational functioning of the individual. In fact, some people with mild mental illness may experience an episode only once. Many people with mild mental illness do not need to be hospitalized, and they often receive psychological and/or medical treatment in the community. The focus of case management in this sense can be about cure. Upon receiving medications and counseling from a mental health worker, the person may completely recover from his or her illness. The likelihood of the majority of individuals with mild mental illness to rely continuously on psychiatric rehabilitation services is relatively low.

Case example. Miss Q was a twenty-four-year-old woman who had finally decided to move out of an abusive relationship four months prior to seeing me. She was diagnosed as having post-traumatic stress disorder. She suffered from horrible nightmares, constantly having dreams about her boyfriend chasing after her with a knife. She experienced panic attacks and slept poorly. She began to have difficulty concentrating on her work, and felt her performance deteriorating. She mentioned in the interviews that her boyfriend had repeatedly abused her physically for the two years they were living together. He continued threatening her with violence after she moved out. Interventions focused on monitoring her mental state; helping her to talk about her experiences; working through some of her anguish, guilt, and low mood; and developing concrete plans to deal with the intruding behaviors of her boyfriend. In addition to counseling, she was also initially put on anti-depressant and antianxiolytic medications. By the sixth month of treatment, she had worked through her issues and terminated her counseling service with me.

A mental health worker takes on different roles and functions when working with people suffering from mild mental illness. The most salient function is one of therapy and counseling. The worker helps the client work through any psychological issues troubling his or her client. However, it is not uncommon for the client to be receiving medications while he or she is seeing the worker. Therefore, assessing and monitoring the mental state of a client are also important functions performed by the mental health worker. Relatively speaking, the worker performs fewer linkage and advocacy functions for a client with mild mental illness than for a client with chronic mental illness.

This critique of the available mental health services brings to light the contexts and constraints of practicing case management. A case manager must understand these constraints, or he or she cannot function effectively within a rather complex mental health care system. This chapter has also introduced two broad target groups for clinical case management: those with chronic and those with mild mental illness. Major differences in assessment and intervention exist for these two target populations. These differences will be further illustrated in Chapters 4 through 7.

Chapter 2

Theoretical Framework
of Clinical Case Management:
A Biopsychosocial
Vulnerability-Stress Perspective

INTRODUCTION

Case Study: Chan Siu Wai

Chan Siu Wai, who lives in a halfway house, is a nineteen-year-old young adult suffering from schizophrenia. His parents are in their forties, and his mother lives in a nearby housing development. He has a younger brother (thirteen years old) and a younger sister (eleven years old) who are living at home with their mother. Currently, he is undergoing prevocational training at a close-by day hospital. Mr. Chan is a taxi driver. Mrs. Chan is also diagnosed with schizophrenia, and is receiving follow-up treatment at an outpatient clinic. However, she is mentally unstable and experiences constant auditory hallucinations. She is argumentative and emotionally labile, and gets into arguments with Siu Wai all the time. Not withstanding this, the two are emotionally attached. For instance, regardless of rain or shine, Siu Wai spends at least two to three hours a day at home during weekdays and almost all days on the weekends while he is living at the halfway house. In the two years prior to living in the halfway house, he had had multiple relapses. The hospital staff suspected that this was due to his enmeshed relationship with his mother. In my interviews with Siu Wai, it became clear that he was caught in a dilemma. On the one hand, he felt that he had to help his mother and protect her. On the other hand, he distasted the emotional climate that mother brought to the family and felt that he did not have any room to think about himself. He is often caught in a flight-or-fight situation with his mother.

Siu Wai experienced his first psychotic episode at the age of fifteen when he heard voices commenting that he was not a good child and student. He also felt that his classmates talked behind his back and constantly looked down on him because he was an immigrant, having left his mother to come live with his father. During a heated argument with a fellow classmate, he punched the student and was brought to the emergency unit of a nearby hospital. Siu Wai came from Fukien at the age of ten. He spoke Fukienese and did not know Cantonese. Moreover, he was brought up by his mother and came to live his father after a ten-year separation. As he said, "I hardly knew my father." Although Siu Wai was now able to communicate fluently in Cantonese, he did not seem to have developed enough social skills to relate to others. He often engaged in very childlike behaviors and had temper tantrums at will. He simply did not realize the normative behaviors that were expected of him in different social situations.

Siu Wai quit school at a young age and had been in and out of the hospitals since then. His educational attainment reached Form 2 standard (eighth grade). However, he liked drawing and seemed to be talented in this area. He was often praised by others for his artistic talent. He aspired to become an artist, but felt he could never do so because of his illness. He tried to resume formal studies. Unfortunately, he could not cope with the stress and thus experienced a few psychotic episodes. Hospital staff suggested that, despite medications, Siu Wai could easily succumb to the stresses of daily life.

It is difficult to say whether Siu Wai clearly understood and accepted his illness. He seemed to understand that some of his experiences were unusual, but did not fully realize the impact of this illness on his overall functioning. Although he had been compliant with medications, he often thought that he would soon be well and did not need them. He disliked attending day hospital, and wanted to start full-time clerical work. As he said to us, "I like to work in the office. I can earn a living and pay my school fees for my art training in the evening." Although this is certainly a noble thought, it would take quite some time before Siu Wai could achieve this. Indeed, Siu Wai was ambivalent about this aspiration himself. He said himself, "People like us [with mental illness] can't make it."

Socially, Siu Wai had a very small circle of friends: one from the hospital and another from the halfway house. He had stopped seeing his classmates since he quit school, and mentioned that he did not want to see them again because "they know I have mental illness." He does not participate much in the activities of the halfway house or day hospital. He usually spends time drawing, and not interacting much with others. As suggested, he has a too-attached relationship with his mother, and a very distant relationship with his father. Moreover, he does not seem to have developed close relationships with his siblings.

How should we conceptualize the issues faced by Chan Siu Wai? Many different factors appear to be affecting his rehabilitation. To begin with, he does not seem to have realistic appraisal and expectations of his rehabilitation. Second, his family environment, particularly his mother, seems to create stress for him, resulting in his relapses. Third, his levels of social and vocational skills are not conducive to his rehabilitation. Last, he lacks the self-confidence to achieve his rehabilitation goals. What framework should we use to organize and make sense of this diverse information? This chapter introduces the bio-psychosocial perspective as the overriding theoretical framework for understanding and working with people with mental illness. Using this perspective, we will delineate the different relevant theories and approaches that are useful for analyzing the conditions faced by a person with mental health problems. These approaches include: vulnerability-stress model, behavioral model, social skills training model, cognitive-behavioral model, and emotion-focused therapy. Means of coping with stress from family and interpersonal relationships within a biopsychosocial perspective will also be discussed.

BIOPSYCHOSOCIAL PERSPECTIVE

A biopsychosocial perspective proposes that biological factors, psychological factors, and social factors affect and are affected by a person's health (Sarafino, 2002). In the case of Chan Siu Wai, biological factors such as heredity may have played a role in influencing the cause and course of his illness. Psychological factors such as a lack of confidence and understanding of illness, and unrealistic expectations and appraisal of his own ability affected Siu Wai's commitment toward his rehabilitation. Socially, Siu Wai's family climate and poor interpersonal relationships are factors that create an impact on his rehabilitation process. This chapter introduces readers to the three sets of factors that influence the cause and course of a person's illness conditions. The specific types of factors are discussed in the following sections.

Biological Factors

Two major subfactors fall under the category of biological factors. These include (1) the genetic materials and processes by which certain characteristics are inherited from our parents, and (2) the biochemical materials that influence the functioning of particular parts of the brain. It has been hypothesized that certain genes are associated with the development of certain types of mental illness. Likewise, it has been suggested that certain biochemical substances called neurotransmitters are related to the development of certain types of mental illness. Essentially, the body is made up of enormously complex physical and biochemical systems. Any defects in the systems and their processes can affect the effective and efficient functioning of these systems, leading to physical and psychosocial dysfunctions. For example, it has been mentioned that the excessive secretion of dopamine, a type of neurotransmitter, has been associated with the positive symptoms experienced by persons suffering from schizophrenia. Indeed, certain types of mental illness may be more strongly influenced by biological factors than others.

Psychological Factors

The psychological makeups of an individual consist of cognition, emotion, and motivation (Sarafino, 2002). *Cognition* is a mental activity that involves processes in perceiving, believing, remembering, and interpreting external events. How an event is perceived, believed, and interpreted will have an enormous impact on the judgment of the individual toward that event, leading to action that is consistent with the judgment and conclusion. For instance, a person who perceives the world, the future, and oneself negatively may feel hopeless and useless, resulting in the experience of depression.

Emotion affects and is affected by one's thoughts, behavior, and physiology. Emotions can be negative or positive, excessive or restricted, and appropriate or inappropriate. For example, when a person is confronted with a stressful life event, he or she feels anxious and experiences palpitations, hot flashes, and other physiological responses. His or her anxieties may also trigger flight-or-fight behavioral responses. Yet, these anxieties may induce a sense of uncontrollability, leading to an overestimation of the threat and harm engendered by the event. In turn, the person becomes even more anxious. In the long run, a person with prolonged exposure to anxieties will develop physical and/or mental health problems.

Motivation is a term that describes why people behave the way they do. In other words, motivation explains why people initiate an action, choose a certain course by which to achieve the action, then persist in doing it. A person's motivation can be affected by his or her cognition and emotions. For instance, a person who does not expect a positive outcome from his or her behavior will not perform enthusiastically. Moreover, when a person is feeling depressed, he or she does not have the motivation to do anything. It is important to note that cognition, emotions, and motivations interact and influence one another. To further complicate the matter, these psychological factors also interact with the biological and social factors, resulting in a certain health status of an individual.

Social Factors

Essentially, social factors include two major subfactors: interpersonal relationship factors and environmental factors. Interpersonal relationships in the family, at work, and with friends can be a source of either stress or support for any individual. Studies (e.g., Cohen & Wills, 1985) have repeatedly suggested that the perceived availability of social support can enhance an indivudual's psychological health and reduce his or her stress level. Interpersonal relationships influence the way a person perceives, behaves, and feels. For example, peer influence has been cited as a reason for taking illicit drugs among young people in different parts of the world. Thus, a person's social behavior can be seen as a product of an interaction between his or her internal and interpersonal processes.

On the environmental level, societal and cultural values affect how a person sees and behaves as well. Psychiatric stigma is one example of an influential environmental factor. A strong stigma is attached to mental illness in Hong Kong and it is closely related to both societal and cultural values held by Chinese people in Hong Kong. As a consequence, persons with mental illness have been socially disadvantaged. For example, people with mental illness have been regarded by prospective employers to be the least preferred employees, and these employers would not select them for interviews (Pearson et al., 2003). Furthermore, social policy also has an impact on the health of individuals. One particular aspect concerns the availability and accessibility of services. Stringent criteria and the lack of resources cause long delays in receiving various general and mental health services in public hospitals in Hong Kong. As a consequence, the health status and the quality of life of individuals has been affected.

It should not be difficult for readers to understand how biological, psychological, and social factors influence the health conditions of an individual. However, the theoretical models described in the following section link these three factors together in a more meaningful way, particularly for understanding mental illness.

BIOPSYCHOSOCIAL THEORIES AND APPROACHES
FOR TREATING MENTAL ILLNESS

Vulnerability-Stress Model

The vulnerability-stress model provides a hypothesis in the understanding of the interactive effects of biological and psychosocial stress factors (Yank, Bentley, & Hargrove, 1993). The two basic factors that influence in this model are described in the following sections.

Biological Factors

This model suggests that genetic or biological factors create different levels of vulnerability in different individuals. Due to the presence of certain genetic or biological dispositions, some people have a lower stress threshold than others, and consequently are more susceptible to developing mental illness. For example, it has been found that people suffering from schizophrenia have a higher level of dopamine (a kind of neurotransmitter) than the general population, and that their bodies emit more dopamine than the receptors in the brain can accommodate, thus accounting for the occurrence of positive symptoms such as hallucinations. This excessive dopamine level also affects the cognitive functioning of an individual with schizophrenia. In essence, the person is unable to process the incoming stimulus, select the appropriate information, derive a plan of actions, and to carry out the action plan. Thus, persons with schizophrenia are biologically vulnerable due to the presence of these genetic predispositions. However, the degree of vulnerability is different for different people.

Psychosocial Factors

According to Yank et al. (1993), psychosocial factors interact with basic vulnerability factors to influence the development of mental illness, such as schizophrenia. It must be stated that not all people with a high level of vulnerability will develop a mental illness, and that individuals with a low level of vulnerability can develop mental illness. Such a difference is due to the amount of psychosocial stress experienced by the individuals. In fact, a person with a high stress threshold may still develop schizophrenia because he or she is confronted with a level of stress higher than even his or her body can withstand. Indeed, only when a person's stress level is above and beyond his or her stress threshold will he or she develop a mental illness. Generally speaking, people with a lower stress threshold are more susceptible to developing a mental illness. Thus, any slight change in individuals' psychosocial conditions can produce stress that crosses their stress threshold and trigger a mental illness.

This model has many strengths. First, it provides a conceptual link between biological, psychological, and social factors in the development of mental illness, and outlines how such development requires the interplay among these three factors. Second, the model focuses interventions on these three factors as well. However, this model has several weaknesses. First, although this model has mentioned such terms as personal protectors and personal risk factors, it fails to spell out clearly the sets of protectors and risk factors that may be related to the development of mental illness. Indeed, this model provides a relatively broad and clear framework, but requires the readers and practitioners to fill in the missing pieces. As well, this model may be criticized for putting a bit too much emphasis on the biological over the social and psychological factors in the causation and treatment of mental illness.

In order to fill in the "missing pieces" and strengthen the psychosocial aspects of this model, it is necessary to incorporate other psychosocial models into this broad stress-vulnerability framework. The rest of the chapter is devoted to this endeavor. Whereas the vulnerability factor can be explained by the biochemical imbalance and other genetic predispositions, psychosocial stress factors can be revealed through an array of psychosocial models, which include: behavioral model, social skills training model, cognitive-behavioral model, and emotion-focused therapy. It must be stated that no one single model can fully explain the causes and course of a person's mental illness. Nor is this an exhaustive list of models. The aforementioned approaches are the major models that have been suggested in the literature (see Table 2.1).

Behavioral Model

Behavior refers to actions (or a lack thereof) performed by an individual in a given social situation. It is a means of relating to another

TABLE 2.1. Developing a Biopsychosocial Vulnerability-Stress Model of Mental Illness

	Biological	Psychological	Social
Vulnerability factors	Genetic and bio-chemical disposi-tions	Cognitive distortions, cognitive rigidity (Cognitive-behav-ioral models)	Lack of social sup-port
		Excessive, inappro-priate, and lack of performance of be-haviors (Behavioral model)	Self-stigma (Con-cept of stigma)
		Problems in skills performance (Social skills training model)	
		Excessive, inappro-priate, and lack of expression of emo-tions; lack of congru-ence in emotions (Emotion-focused therapy)	
Environmental stress factor			Family stress (Expressed emo-tions)
			Stress from interper-sonal relationship
			Social stigma

human being. However, inadequate, inappropriate, and excessive behavioral performances affect our interaction with others, leading to negative consequences. Indeed, people with mental illness manifest different behavioral problems, such as excessive and inappropriate behaviors (e.g., odd mannerisms) or inadequate behaviors (e.g., a lack of self-care skills). These behavioral problems are due to vulnerability factors that constrain the person's responses to external psychosocial stresses.

The behavioral model emphasizes the importance of learning to distinguish normal and abnormal behaviors, and suggests that mental health problems are related to learning maladaptive behaviors through a process of classical and/or operant conditioning (Martin & Pear, 1999). According to this model, different learning principles, such as positive and negative reinforcements and positive and negative punishments account for the acquisition of abnormal behaviors in a person. This model also maintains that changes in behaviors will lead to the changes in a person's cognition and emotions. Thus, it is important to identify the problem behaviors and to derive different learning principles for the acquisition of alternative and new behaviors.

According to the ABC concept of the behavioral model, A is the antecedent, B stands for behaviors, and C is the consequences. Although it is important to quantify a problem behavior so that it is measurable and observable, it is equally important to examine how the consequences of the behaviors have strengthened the reoccurrence of the behavior. One must examine the different learning principles underneath the performance of such a behavior.

Case Example: Gary

Gary is a fifty-six-year-old man, living alone, suffering from panic disorder and agoraphobia. He has been keeping himself at home for the past several months after having been badly assaulted by a burglar. Gary used to be a rather active and sociable person. It looks as though this traumatic event has clearly changed his lifestyle and behaviors. Using the behavioral model to analyze Gary's problem, it is apparent that this incident has created many anxieties and fears for Gary. He is so fearful and insecure that he dares not go out of his house. This avoidance behavior invariably soothes his anxieties and fears. Therefore, whenever he begins to feel anxious and fearful about having to leave the house, he avoids these anxieties and fears by simply not going out. Consequently, he becomes socially withdrawn. In keeping with the behavioral model, it is necessary for Gary to be desensitized of this fear by gradually and systematically going out of the house.

This behavioral model may also be useful in understanding the situations of people with depression and schizophrenia. In the case of people with depression, it is always useful to plan to gradually increase their activity level. Moreover, the depressed mood of individuals with depression may be gradually lifted by exploring and enhancing the activities they deem pleasurable. People with schizophrenia can also benefit a great deal from the behavioral model of treatment. It has been argued that people with chronic schizophrenia suffer from severe cognitive deficits. As a result, they have lost many skills essential for daily living. Therefore, behavioral programs can be designed to help these individuals regain those skills. Indeed, skills training has become an important part of the overall treatment goals for people with chronic schizophrenia. In the literature, skills training includes such areas as social and problem-solving skills, self-care skills, domestic-living skills, community-living skills, money management, leisure and job seeking, and job-related skills. Workers need to assess these skills areas and derive from them behavioral programs to train individuals to acquire these skills. Along with individual training programs, token economy (rewarding patients for appropriate behaviors with tokens that they can exchange for various prizes) has been widely used in the psychiatric services to help clients relearn certain skills and behaviors.

In general, it is necessary for mental health workers to examine the behaviors of people with mental health problems. Although behaviors may sometimes be the main focus of intervention, they can also be considered simply as an initial entry point for changing other aspects of a person's overall conditions. Adopting a behavioral model as part of the treatment modalities offers several advantages. First, this model attempts to specify behaviors and problems in very concrete terms, and, therefore, demystify the therapeutic process. Moreover, when it is planned with sufficient detail, people with little professional training can administer the procedures. Third, clients with a certain degree of cognitive deficits can also benefit from this treatment model. However, this model ignores other factors such as cognition and emotions, when determining abnormal behaviors. Moreover, workers may become too technical in applying the various procedures and disregard the humanness that is an important element of the therapeutic process.

Social Skills Training Model

Liberman, Neuchterlein, & Wallace (1982) have provided a theoretical framework for incorporating social skills training into the vulnerability-stress model of schizophrenia. Essentially, they identified a number of critical stress and vulnerability factors that are closely related to the performance of social skills by people with schizophrenia. These include psychosocial stress factors such as interpersonal communication in the family and the amount of life stresses encountered, and vulnerability factors such as the severity of symptoms suffered by the person, motivation deficits, and cognitive deficits. *Interpersonal communication* refers to the problematic communication between family members, friends, co-workers, and acquaintences and the person with schizophrenia. It is suggested that a stressful family and interpersonal climate may lead to relapses for the person with schizophrenia. Motivational and cognitive deficits adversely affect how a person with schizophrenia defines a problem, selects relevant information in the interpersonal situations, understands social mores, and chooses an appropriate course of responses in social interactions. Indeed, a person with schizophrenia suffering from motivational and cognitive deficits will not be socially skilled to perform in many social situations. They tend to have difficulty resolving the problems of daily life. As Liberman et al. (1982) put it, "It is possible that schizophrenics, because of their perceptual and cognitive impairments, and increased psychological vulnerability, are stressed by mundane, small scale and everyday life events that would not be upsetting to normals" (p. 14).

As a consequence, people with schizophrenia tend to avoid stressful social interactions or are unable to interact properly with people around them. Therefore, it is useful to provide social skills training for individuals with schizophrenia so that they can develop competence to handle environment stresses, thus reducing the possibility of relapses. However, Liberman et al. (1982) challenged the traditional social skills training program for "bypassing the more critical psychological processes that are closely linked with attention, perception, and information processing" (p. 40). They found that social skills training that focuses only on the topographical features of social skills—eye contact, gestures, voice volume, assertive responses—may lead to limited generalization, partially because the cognitive processes that facilitate many different types of social behaviors in different situations are not targeted in treatment. Thus, it is important to include cognitive precursors of social skills, such as problem definition, accurate perception of relevant information in interpersonal situations, knowledge of social mores, and ability to choose an appropriate course of response, in social skills training.

Demonstrable effects show that social skills training improves the social and occupational functioning of people with schizophrenia (Cook & Razzano, 2000; Tsang & Pearson, 2001). On a broader perspective, social skills training has been an important driving force toward a skills training approach in working with people with chronic schizophrenia. With the loss of the basic and requisite skills for living, individuals with schizophrenia have to be retrained to regain such skills as domestic-living skills, transportation, self-care, community-living skills, etc. In Hong Kong, many community rehabilitation services include a skills training component as one of the treatment modalities for persons with schizophrenia. Therefore, mental health workers should learn to incorporate the social skills training model in assessing and working with people with mental illness.

However, the behavioral model and social skills training model cannot adequately address an individual's lack of motivation to perform certain behaviors or stop behaving in certain ways. One must draw on the cognitive model to find the answers.

Cognitive-Behavioral Model

Social learning theory suggests that people do not necessarily learn certain behaviors through classical and operant conditioning but learn through a cognitive process of observation and modeling. Cognitive theorists have ventured even further and suggest that cognition plays a vital role in determining whether a person can learn and unlearn certain behaviors. Indeed, they believe that human behavioral and emotional problems are directly related to how a person views the world and responds to it accordingly. It is not difficult for mental health workers to realize that many clients have a lifelong pattern of distorted or irrational thinking, and that they are more prone to interpret situations negatively and incorrectly. Thus, these malfunctioning cognitive processes intensify a person's stressful experiences and lower his or her stress threshold.

Different cognitive models suggest different cognitive processes that account for the problems in the human mind. For example, rational emotive behavior therapy (REBT) maintains that people rigidly holding such irrational beliefs as "Everything I do must be absolutely perfect, otherwise I am a failure" and "life is fair" would be unhappy because they have high and unshakable expectations about others and themselves (Ellis, 1993). As a consequence, they feel unhappy when their expectations are unfulfilled (Ellis, 1986). Cognitive behavior modification (CBM) is another cognitive-behavioral therapy, proposed by Meichenbaum (1986). This therapy aims at changing a person's self-verbalization from negative self-talk to positive self-talk. For change to occur, the person needs to be aware of and able to interrupt his or her negative self-talk before it leads to dysfunctional behaviors and thinking. The person must learn to engage in positive self-talk as a means to practice adaptive coping skills for his or her problems. Some people rename this therapy "coping skills training."

Beck (1979) introduces another cognitive-behavioral model called cognitive therapy. This therapy states that the way people feel and behave is determined by how they perceive and structure their experiences. It is an insight-oriented therapy that emphasizes recognizing and changing negative thoughts and maladaptive beliefs. According to Beck (1995), three fundamental cognitive contents are related to the development of emotional problems: (1) automatic thoughts, (2) intermediate beliefs, and (3) core beliefs. *Automatic thoughts* refer to reflexive self-statements or images that an individual involuntarily experiences throughout daily life. These statements and images can be distorted from reality, and are then classified under different types of cognitive distortions such as absolutist thoughts, arbitrary inferences, and overgeneralizations. Essentially, an individual experiencing negative automatic thoughts misinterprets a situation and negatively distorts its reality. This distorted interpretation is heavily influenced by the person's schema, which includes both intermediate beliefs and core beliefs. *Intermediate beliefs* are rules, assumptions, and attitudes a person holds. *Core beliefs* are a person's underlying, foundational beliefs that influence both intermediate beliefs and automatic thoughts. For example, if a person appraises himself or herself as inadequate, he or she may hold such rules and assumptions as "Whatever I have accomplished is because someone else has made it possible" and "No matter how hard I try, I can never make it." An individual having these intermediate beliefs may experience different types of cognitive distortions (automatic thoughts). If an employer comments negatively on the individual's performance on a certain task, he or she may remark, "I have made a complete mess of the situation," even if the reality is that he or she has made only a small mistake but has otherwise completed the task smoothly and on time (selective abstraction). According to Beck (1995), core beliefs influence one's intermediate beliefs and automatic thoughts. Moreover, these cognitive contents affect how a person behaves and feels. Using the previous example again, since the employee thinks he or she has made a mess of the situation, the individual feels very disappointed and shameful and avoids making contact with colleagues and bosses.

Cognitive-behavioral models clearly highlight the importance of cognitive contents in influencing the mental health of individuals. In the literature, it has been found that cognitive therapy has been particularly effective in helping people with depression and anxiety disorders. Moreover, it has also been widely used in treating people with personality disorders. In schizophrenia, cognitive therapy has been tried on people with severe positive symptoms. It is necessary to include the cognitive-behavioral models in the assessment and treatment for people with different mental disorders. Including cognitive aspects in assessing and working with people with mental illness offers several advantages. First, research has clearly revealed that cognition plays a part in shaping a person's normal and abnormal behaviors, and, therefore, is undoubtedly a potential area of intervention. Second, cognitive-behavioral strategies have been used with some success in dealing with people with different mental health problems. However, clinical experiences show that people who do not possess a certain level of cognitive competence may not benefit from this line of intervention. Quite often, these individuals do not understand or have difficulty self-examining their own cognitive processes. In addition, people who are overwhelmed with emotions do not seem to benefit from a cognitive therapy because, at this particular moment in time, they need to deal with their emotional rather than cognitive problems.

Emotion-Focused Therapies

Emotion is an integral part of a person's personality. It affects and is affected by one's thoughts, behavior, and physiology. Negative, excessive, restricted, or inappropriate emotions are signs and symptoms of different types of mental health problems. For example, whereas depression is characterized by excessively low moods and negative emotions such as guilt and self-blame, anxiety problems are expressed through excessive worries and fear. However, a person's inability to fully and freely express his or her emotions and achieve a sense of congruence between emotions, behavior, and cognition is often described as the underlying reason for his or her emotional and mental health problems. Indeed, emotional problems can paralyze an individual from being able to withstand stressful environmental conditions, thus serving as vulnerability factors to the individual.

Different types of emotion-focused therapies attempt to help people understand and develop strategies to handle their emotions. Gestalt therapy, person-centered therapy, play therapy, and existential therapy are among the most commonly known intervention models using the humanistic perspective. Take person-centered therapy, for example. This therapy was developed by Carl Rogers (Rogers, 1961). Several basic assumptions can be made about this therapy. To begin with, humans have an innate tendency toward self-actualization and to become fully functioning people. Unfortunately, since childhood, we live under many conditions that are set by others. We conform to these conditions because we want to be loved and approved by people who are significant to us. As a consequence, we ignore our own needs and deny our inner feelings and wishes. In Rogerian terms, we live under situations of conditional worth and have become more and more alienated from our ideal self, living in the real self that represents only a facade for others. Emotional problems occur when a person experiences incongruence between his or her ideal and the real selves.

Another important assumption of this therapy is that "significant positive personality change does not occur except in relationship" (Rogers, 1980). Thus, it is paramount for a worker to create a therapeutic relationship that creates a positive psychological atmosphere in which the client can experience his or her inner feelings and wishes. According to Rogers, at least three characteristics exist in this type of relationship: unconditional positive regard, empathetic understanding, and genuineness/congruence. As Rogers (1961) claims, these characteristics are necessary and sufficient to facilitate a client's personality changes.

Existential therapy views our human existence as ever evolving and a continual re-creation of ourselves through meaningful activities (Yalom, 1980). By engaging in such activities, we find meaning in our existence. Essentially, this therapy suggests that although we do not have a choice regarding what had happened in our past, we have a choice what we want to be. Moreover, this therapy maintains that we have the capacity for self-awareness: to understand that we have freedom as well as responsibility for ourselves; that we are alone and yet striving to relate to others in a meaningful way; and that we are on a constant search for meaning, values, and goals in order to ascertain our existence. This therapy also predicates that because of our capacity for self-awareness, we are inevitably confronted with existential anxieties. These anxieties stem from the feelings of aloneness, freedom to choose our future, and knowing that we are responsible for ourselves. One of the main goals of this therapy is to help a client become aware of his or her restricted existence, which is often characterized by limited choices and existential anxiety and unhappiness. Furthermore, the worker will encourage the client to take action to change his or her life.

These models share a few things in common: (1) they provide a platform for individuals to express and experience their emotions; (2) they help individuals become aware of their emotions as well as how attitudes, behaviors, and life circumstances have contributed to the development of their emotional disturbances; (3) these therapies assume that when people are aware of their emotions and underlying issues, they will be free to choose among alternatives, thus shaping their own destiny; and (4) workers need to create a therapeutic relationship that can help clients explore their own self.

Emotions constitute an important part of the overall assessment and intervention for people with mental health problems. Particularly, emotions becomes an essential intervention focus when individuals are overwhelmed by certain emotions (e.g., grief reaction). Unless individuals have sufficient time and space for expressing their emotions, they will be unable to engage in any self-exploration or to work on any personal issues. Furthermore, central to the humanistic perspective, emotions are the means to gain further and deeper self-understanding. With self-understanding, these individuals can then realize their own inner experiences and make choices for themselves. Consequently, they shall enjoy a fuller functioning and achieve a greater degree of self-actualization. In other words, they achieve better mental health. As well, managing emotions is also part of the intervention focus. Since excessive or inadequate expression of emotions may be detrimental to clients' health, mental health workers often need to teach clients the necessary skills for managing their emotions. Moreover, the ability to manage one's emotions creates a sense of efficacy.

Social Factors

Four concepts are frequently mentioned in the literature to explain how interpersonal and environmental factors influence an individual's mental health: family stress, social support, stress from social relationships, and stigma. These factors influence mental health by being either environmental stressors or environmental protectors. Individuals who are exposed to excessive and prolonged environmental stressors that exceed their coping abilities are susceptible to developing mental illness. Conversely, environmental protectors buffer the stresses experienced by the individuals. The literature offers few concepts relating to the social and environmental factors that influence the cause and course of development of mental illness.

Family Stress

Expressed emotions as a family communication problem can be viewed as a possible environmental stressor that influences the development of mental illness. This concept has been given much attention in the past thirty years. Expressed emotions denote a high degree of closeness and high emotional reactivity and intensity in a family. Inadequate problem solving and conflict resolution skills of a family are also implied in this concept. Family stress suggests that dysfunctional family communication patterns, which include critical comments, emotional overinvolvement, and hostility, are associated with relapses in persons with schizophrenia. (This will be further elaborated in Chapter 8.) Research findings have repeatedly found that the mentally ill relatives whose family members had high scores in critical comments, emotional overinvolvement, and hostility, called high expressed emotions (HEE), had a much greater chance of relapse than those whose family scored low in these areas, or had low expressed emotions (LEE). Thus, the amount of expressed emotions in a family serves as environmental stressor for people with mental illness.

Family stress can occur on the other side as well. In the literature, it is found that family members suffer from burdens and poor physical and mental health as a result of taking continuous care of their relatives with serious mental illness (Hatfield & Lefley, 1993). They have to handle practical difficulties, such as the lack of understanding of the causes of illnesses, of treatment, and of the mental health systems; as well as relating to the day-to-day management of their relatives with mental illness. Consequently, many experience psychological and social costs associated with the caregiving burdens. Examples of psychological costs are anxieties, frustrations, worries, guilt, grief, fear, and anger toward having a relative suffering from serious mental illness. An increase in family conflicts, limited friendship and social networks, financial difficulties, and a change in daily routine are examples of social costs associated with the care of a relative with mental illness. Since it can be frustrating and distressing to take care of a person with mental illness, family members may respond to their relatives with negativism and at times indifference, thus leading to an intense family climate that is stress inducing for all involved. On the contrary, family members who are supportive of their relatives may provide them with the necessary buffers against environmental stresses.

Looking at it from a vulnerability-stress perspective, although family members can inadvertently become a source of environmental stress for their relatives with mental illness, they can also play an important role in the successful rehabilitation of their relatives. Mental health workers need to understand how family dynamics affect the mental health of individuals with mental illness.

Social Support

Literature suggests that adequate social support promotes better physical and mental health and enhances stress-coping abilities. Social support helps to redefine the severity of the impending stressful events by reassuring the person that he or she will have someone to help him or her in times of difficulties as well as resources on which to draw to solve their problems (Walsh, 2000). The first point is related to a perception of the availability of social support, and the second point is concerned with the actual provision of support. In general, the literature suggests that social networks provide emotional support, social companionship, and information to individuals. Moreover, it is generally agreed upon that the larger one's social network, the more the sources of social support.

On the other hand, the lack of social support can become a vulnerability factor for individuals with mental illness. This should not be difficult to understand because individuals without adequate social support do not have strong buffers against environmental stressors (i.e., they lack emotional support, a successful means of gaining information, and companionship). Coupled with the cognitive deficits that seriously affect illness suffers' problem-solving abilities, these individuals are particularly vulnerable to experiencing relapses during times of difficulty. Thus, it is useful to study the concept of social support to facilitate an understanding of social stress factors in the course and cause of development of mental illness.

Stress from Social Relationships

Social relationship difficulties are stress inducing for people with mental illness. Intense conflicts or indifference at work within friendship circles can generate stress for people with mental illness and can reduce their network size, thus limiting the availability of social support. Since individuals with severe mental illness are particularly sensitive to environmental stressors, social relationship problems that are bearable for other people may be unbearable for illness suffers. Moreover, they do not have adequate social and problem-solving skills that help them resolve these social relationship problems. As a result, people with severe mental illness are vulnerable to experiencing relapses.

It is important to include the concept of stress from social relationships in the assessment and intervention for people with mental health problems. Social relationships can serve as both environmental protectors and stresses for people with mental illness. Workers must assess clearly whether the social networks surrounding a person with a mental illness are stress buffering or stress inducing. Workers should not assume that the networks are necessarily supportive. They also need to decide whether they would help the person get connected to a certain network or would rather help the person to disengage from it. Each person is different and must be assessed individually. Moreover, supportive and unsupportive ties change over time and must be reassessed periodically. Nonetheless, as Walsh (2000) asserts, mental health workers should help persons with mental illness develop informal supportive networks as much as it is possible.

Stigma

Two relevant concepts about psychiatric stigma exist: social stigma and self-stigma. The former refers to social prejudice held toward persons with mental illness. These individuals are labeled and treated negatively by the general public. For example, persons with mental illness are discriminated by employers and colleagues at work. A study conducted by Pearson et al. (2003) found that prospective employers were least inclined to offer job interviews to persons with mental disability. People with developmental and physical handicaps, on the other hand, were given more opportunities for job interviews. Essentially, the general public harbors the misconception that people with mental illness are dangerous and are prone to exhibit violent behaviors. As a consequence, people with mental illness experience stress and discrimination generated from neighbors, employers, friends, relatives, and family members.

Self-stigma refers to the degree to which an individual accepts the socially and negatively prescribed label of mentally ill (Hayward & Bright, 1997). People with a strong self-stigma are extremely uncomfortable to have their "identities" revealed to others. They also try very hard to conceal their identities. Others appear to have very low self-esteem and passively accept a marginalized and depleted lifestyle. Indeed, they may acquire a strong sense of powerlessness and may become unmotivated to change in their lives. As a consequence, these individuals do not respond positively and actively toward rehabilitative treatment.

Thus, stigma can be perceived as an environmental stress and vulnerability factor. It is a stress factor because people in the environment may be hostile and unfriendly toward those with mental illness, thus inducing stress onto these individuals. It is a vulnerability factor because people with mental illness who have acquired self-stigma are overwhelmed by a sense of powerlessness and passivity. When they are faced with stressful situations, they may not actively engage in productive problem-solving activities. Eventually, this may lead to their psychiatric relapses. As mental health workers, we need to include the concept of stigma in the overall conceptual framework for understanding the situations faced by people with mental illness.

CONCLUSION

A number of concluding remarks can be generated from this framework:

1. No model exists that can clearly and comprehensively explain the causes and conditions of mental illness.
2. Different models emphasize certain aspects of a person's condition that influence the cause and course of his or her mental ill-

ness. Thus, the concepts and ideas of different models need to be utilized to comprehend the situation of a person with mental illness. Indeed, different models interact to provide a clearer understanding of the person's situation.

3. In conclusion, mental health workers ought to be familiarized with these various explanatory and intervention models so that they can draw on the concepts and ideas to understand the conditions of their clients with mental illness. Moreover, some of these models have clear descriptions of the assessment and intervention strategies and skills for helping individuals with mental illness. Workers can draw on these intervention strategies and skills in working with people with mental illness.

Chapter 3

Psychiatric Assessment

INTRODUCTION

The overall objective of a comprehensive psychiatric assessment is for a mental health worker to understand the profile of a person with a mental disorder and then, based on the profile, work with the client to formulate his or her rehabilitation goals. It is an important part of the case management process because the formulated goals provide direction for both the client and the case manager. These goals also serve as the baseline for evaluating the changes and progress in the client. Psychiatric assessment is different from psychological assessment in that it includes an assessment of the biomedical, psychological, and social conditions of a client. This chapter will critically review the four major models of assessment and will discuss the strengths and limitations of each of these models. It is argued here that no one single model can fully capture the issues faced by persons with mental health problems, and thus a comprehensive psychiatric assessment model for people with mental health problems needs to be developed. The second part of this chapter is devoted to a detailed delineation of a biopsychosocial vulnerability-stress model of psychiatric assessment.

MODELS OF ASSESSMENT

Four assessment models can be used for understanding the mental health conditions of a person with mental illness. They are described in the following sections.

The Medical or Curative Model

The medical model centers on the symptoms of a mental illness, with an understanding that an individual with a cluster of symptoms will be diagnosed with a certain mental disorder based on those symptoms. At present, two major classification systems are used for mental disorders: *Diagnostic and Statistical Manual of Mental Disorders,* Fourth Edition, Text Revision (American Psychiatric Association, 2000) and *ICD-10 Classification of Mental and Behavioral Disorders* (World Health Organization, 1992). These manuals set out the criteria for diagnosing a mental disorder. For example, in depression, the person must exhibit either a depressed mood or a loss of interest along with and five other symptoms including sleep disturbance, change in appetite, and change in weight. Duration of symptoms is another important criterion as well. For example, depressive symptoms must be present for at least two consecutive weeks before the person can be given a diagnostic label of depression.

Several assumptions underlie this medical model. First, it assumes that a biological/genetic basis exists in the etiology of mental illness. For example, people with depression have a lower level of serotonin than the general population, and this lowered level of serotonin is somehow responsible for the occurrence of depression in those individuals. Another assumption is that if an identifiable cause of mental illness exists, a cure exists. Medications become the major therapeutic intervention used in this model.

The medical model makes the following contributions to assessment and interventions in mental illness. First, this model highlights the possible biological (genetic) causes of some kinds of mental illness. For example, it has been suggested that an excessive level of dopamine is strongly associated with the occurrence of positive symptoms found among people with schizophrenia. Indeed, evidence and clinical experiences have shown that certain mental illnesses have a biological or genetic base, and some clients appear to be more strongly affected by biological factors than are others (Kendall & Hammen, 1995).

Second, this model may be reassuring to clients and their family members. Since it is not uncommon to find some family members harboring the thought that they are responsible for causing their relatives' mental illness (Pearson, 1993), this medical or biological model provides the family members and the clients with a perspective that it is not their fault. Indeed, such an occurrence is something beyond their control. Consequently, this reduces the guilt and shame borne by the clients and their family members. Indeed, this view has been adopted by mental health organizations, such as the National Alliance of the Mentally Ill (NAMI, 2004). Another possible advantage of this model is that it may encourage some clients to accept their illnesses and comply with medications. Simply put, people generally believe that medical problems should be treated with medications. If mental illness is seen in the same light, it should be treated accordingly.

Holding too strongly to this medical model presents obvious disadvantages. First, it can be problematic to make a diagnosis based simply on the occurrence of a cluster of symptoms, because the same set of symptoms may have a different cause, and, therefore, can be misdiagnosed as a different type of mental disorder. For instance, a person with hypothyroidism exhibiting depressive symptoms could be misdiagnosed as having depression. Such a misdiagnosis could lead to improper medical treatments for the illness and might also create a labeling effect for the individual. Another possible disadvantage to this model is that medical interventions may lead to undesirable outcomes, such as intolerable side effects of medications and social stigma. With regard to medications, some drugs such as typical antipsychotic medications cause serious side effects that are quite intolerable to some of the clients. For example, chlorpromazine can create drowsiness, dry mouth, constipation, and agitation for some clients. These side effects not only create personal discomfort for some clients, but also affect their social and occupational performance (Hellewell, 2002). As a consequence, some clients refuse to take the medications. This creates problems for mental health workers and family members. Even when the workers and family members acknowledge the necessity of psychotropic medications for those clients who are suffering from such diseases as schizophrenia, they are not always successful in encouraging their clients or relatives to comply with the medications. Indeed, some family members find this to be a constant source of stress and conflicts (Wong, Pui, Pearson, & Chiu, 2003).

One last point about the medical model is that it may create false hope for clients and family members. Medical science often aims to identify and cure diseases, with the belief that if a cause can be identified, a cure can be identified. However, the causes of different types of mental illness have yet to be found or confirmed, and not a single drug can "cure" mental illness. At this stage of the medical development it is generally agreed upon that psychotropic medications can only control the manifestations of symptoms (Bentley, 1998). Undue faith in medical science may create false hope among some clients and family members.

The Disability Model

This model originated from a group of social psychiatrists who were treating persons with chronic mental illness (e.g., Wing & Morris, 1981). Two basic assumptions can be made about this model. First, mental illness is a long-term, disabling illness, sometimes with a deteriorating course. As such, psychiatric impairments are associated with mental disorder, and the more severe a person's psychiatric impairments, the more severe his or her disability. Second, people with chronic mental illness require an array of medical, psychological, social, and vocational rehabilitation services to help them travel through their illness. According to Wing and Morris (1981), assessment focuses on the understanding of the impact of psychiatric impairments, social disadvantages, and personal reactions of the individuals.

This model makes substantial contributions to assessment and interventions in mental health. It acknowledges the multiple factors in the environment and in the person that can affect his or her level of psychiatric disability. The disability model encourages multilevel interventions, targeting changes not only at the client's biological functioning but also at his or her psychosocial functioning. This model is graphically depicted in Figure 3.1, with biological factors and psychosocial factors on the two ends of the X axis, and medical interventions and psychosocial interventions on the two ends of the Y axis. This conceptual diagram is useful for placing the different factors affecting the illness and rehabilitation process of a client on the diagram to help the worker determine the corresponding intervention focuses for helping the client.

Another contribution of this model is that it highlights the need for a multidisciplinary team of experts in order to achieve an accurate assessment and treatment of a client with chronic mental illness. Each

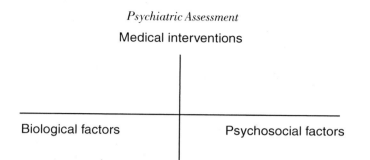

FIGURE 3.1. The Disability Model

discipline provides expert knowledge and skills relating to its area of expertise, and treatment goals and action plans for the client must take into account of the views of the different professionals involved.

Several criticisms can be made about this model. First, this model overemphasizes the client's deficits and disabilities and overlooks his or her potential and strengths. Indeed, undue concerns over deficits and disabilities create dependency and ignore human creativity in addressing problems of living. Disability and illness are overly emphasized in this model, overlooking that such factors form only part of the person's total well-being. Second, although this model provides a framework to examine the biopsychosocial conditions of a client, it does not provide sufficient details to inform clinical practices. Third, this is an expert model and relies mainly on medical and health care professionals to make clinical judgments and decisions. Clients remain passive, and their concerns and aspirations may not always be known by the professionals. Last, disputes over the correct course of treatment often occur among different professionals in the multidisciplinary team meetings. Much time is spent arriving at a compromise.

Skills Model

The skills model maintains that human beings need to acquire certain skills in order to live, learn, and work in the community with the least amount of support (Liberman, Neuchterlein, & Wallace, 1982). This model does not deny the importance of medications in treating persons with mental illness. It claims that medication is necessary, but not sufficient for these individuals. This model stresses the teaching of skills as essential to the independent functioning of the clients in the community. Domestic-living skills, social skills, and community-living skills are some examples (see Appendix I). Such skills are functional in nature and can be unlearned, learned, and relearned.

The skills model has been widely applied in working with people suffering from chronic mental illness. Many of these individuals have severe behavioral deficits and/or excesses, and some of them cannot even perform very simple tasks. In the case of persons with chronic schizophrenia, it has been found that these individuals have serious cognitive deficits. They have difficulty receiving and processing information, deriving action plans, and carrying out the action plans (Liberman et al., 1982). As a consequence, they cannot perform the necessary skills required in diverse social situations. For example, one of my clients suffering from severe auditory hallucinations (voices of an angel and a devil quarreling with one another) was very preoccupied with the voices and could not engage in daily activities and social interactions. He had difficulty receiving and processing relevant information, leading to poor social and vocational skill performances. In the past thirty years, the skills model has been widely incorporated into different rehabilitation programs for people with serious mental illness, and results have suggested that the skills model was effective in improving the level of skills of clients and reducing their relapse rate (Liberman et al., 1982; Trower, Bryant, & Argyle, 1986). In Hong Kong, many halfway houses and day training centers have adopted a skills model as one of the major components in their intervention practices.

The skills model offers three major contributions to assessment and interventions in mental health. First, assessment specifically focuses on understanding the functional skills essential for the individual living in specific social contexts and environments. For example, a client who wants to work as a clerical assistant will be assessed on specific skill requirements related to clerical work, and will be trained to perform the necessary skills. Second, following the behavioral traditions, this model utilizes a specific set of procedures for assessment and treatment. These procedures can be acquired relatively easily and quickly through training. Third, training programs are individualized. Since every client is different, this model provides treatment plans and strategies to suit individual needs.

However, some criticisms can be made about this model. First, it does not distinguish between lacking a skill and lacking motivation to perform the skill. For example, a person who does not work up to his or her ability because he or she knows that doing so would lead to more responsibility has the skills, but does not have the motivation to use them. Second, this is a deficit model and assumes the acquisition of new or appropriate skills to be the ultimate goals of an individual. Although this claim has a grain of truth, it does not take into consideration the subjective personal dimensions such as interests, satisfaction, and quality of life. Indeed, this model appears to encourage a person to fit into a certain prescribed mode of life (i.e., maintaining a status quo), but ignores the personal growth that is possible that can go beyond an individual's personal and environmental constraints. Similarly, this model stresses the acquisition of functional skills and disregards the importance of learning skills for the enjoyment of life.

Strengths Model

Theorists and practitioners such as Cowger (1992) and Rapp (1998b) have criticized the previous models as trying only to help the clients manage symptoms, correct deficits, and, at best, maintain their status quo in a society. Indeed, the previous models appear to have created an illness identity for the individual under which her or she is defined by his or her illness. According to the strengths model proposed by Cowger (1992), successful recovery from a mental illness rests with:

- seeing the illness only as a part of the person;
- having a sense of personal choices and control;
- having a purpose in living;
- experiencing a sense of achievement;
- having supportive relationships; and
- being personally involved in the action of change.

Instead of focusing on personal deficits and problems, this model emphasizes understanding the client's desires, goals, ambitions, and hopes as well as developing his or her internal and external resources to fulfill his or her goals. The worker provides the client with as many choices as possible during the rehabilitation process with the ultimate concern being to give the client a sense of satisfaction and achievement. Another important aspect of this model is that it is paramount that the client is actively involved in the process of change. He or she should make as many decisions as he or she is capable of making, and should see that those decisions and actions have affected his or her well-being. The client is empowered through this process. Research findings reported that the strengths model achieves positive results by improving the quality of life, reducing hospitalization, and improving occupational and vocational functioning (Rapp, 1998a).

Using the case of Ah Lee from Chapter 1, other models would have explored the impacts of psychiatric impairments on Ah Lee's functioning, or would have examined Ah Lee's areas of skill deficits: concentration span, getting a part-time job, getting up earlier in the morning, better drug compliance, etc. However, it would be fruitless to adopt these models with Ah Lee. Unless his self-image improved, he would not have the motivation to change his life circumstances. Indeed, his usual saying was, "I'm nothing. I can do nothing. Just let me stay in bed as long as I want. This is my only enjoyment in life." Changes had to come from him and had to come gradually by tapping into his interests. An opportunity arrived when Ah Lee mentioned that he found some strength after going jogging one day. With his permission, the key worker went jogging with him. Jogging served as a catalyst for Ah Lee to become interested in other activities. He then began playing table tennis and badminton. With the increase in his energy level and successes in winning tennis and badminton (playing against staff and other residents of the halfway house), he became more interested in exploring the possibility of getting a job as a clerical assistant. However, this long-term goal was broken down into short-term goals of learning to increase his concentration span, strategies to cope with his persistent auditory hallucination, skills in clerical work, etc. During the entire process, Ah Lee was encouraged to identify his interests and goals and to participate in making the decisions regarding when and how he would fulfill his goals. My job was to support him in doing these tasks and to help him draw on his internal resources and to link him to outside resources as needed.

The contributions of this model to assessment and interventions in mental health are as follows:

1. This model deemphasizes pathology and deficits and rightly asserts that illness is just part of the whole person. It places emphasis on the strengths of an individual, capitalizing on his or her internal and external resources to foster changes. In assessment and treatment, this model explores internal resources such as aspirations and competencies and external resources such as material resources and the support network of the individual.
2. This model does not see the person as an object of change but as a change agent. He or she is active in the rehabilitation process, making the efforts toward achievement and growth.
3. Finally, similar to the skills model, this model is individualized, and rehabilitation plans and interventions are tailor-made to fit each individual.

Although this model highlights strengths and resources as the focus of assessment and interventions, it may underestimate the impact of mental illness on the lives of an individual. As such, it can create a sense of false hope, leading to frustrations and despair when the aspirations of the client cannot be fulfilled. In fact, external environment constraints restrict an individual's choices. Internally, the psychiatric impairments and adverse personal reactions to illness are strong enough to these constrain the ability of an individual to fulfill his or her aspirations, affecting his or her confidence and competencies. For example, a client who has the goal of getting a full-time job may become frustrated because the job market is poor. Finally, conflict may occur between individual rights and choices and those of the society. For example, a client may refuse to be hospitalized despite being mentally unstable. Undue regard for the client's rights can pose a threat to the safety of others in the society.

Although none of the previously mentioned assessment models can fully capture the dynamic interplay of biopsychosocial factors in influencing the cause and course of development of a person's mental illness, these assessment models point out the following facts, constituting six guiding principles for a good assessment for persons with mental illness:

- Mental illnesses and mental health problems are the results of the interplay among the biological, psychological, and social factors that affect the lives of the individual.
- Identification and development of the strengths of the individual are part and parcel of an accurate assessment and successful interventions.
- Assessment and interventions are eclectic in nature. Different models complement one another.
- Choices of intervention methods depend on the types and severity of the client's illness, his or her preferences, availability of resources, and the worker's own repertoire of skills and resources.
- The worker needs to help the client make the right choice of treatment and to help him or her strike a balance between the right of client and that of others in society.
- Accurate assessment and effective interventions rely on the cooperation and efforts of a multidisciplinary team of experts.

BIOPSYCHOSOCIAL VULNERABILITY-STRESS MODEL OF PSYCHIATRIC ASSESSMENT

This assessment framework is based on a biopsychosocial perspective of health and disease, and normally includes the following areas: (1) medical/physical aspects, (2) social and family aspects, (3) vocational aspects, and (4) psychological aspects. It also incorporates the vulnerability-stress perspective discussed in Chapter 2. In making a psychiatric assessment, it is necessary to explore the various biological, social, and psychological stress and vulnerability factors that affect the life of a client. It is also useful to explore the deficits and strengths found in these areas. Each area should contain strengths and deficits that help or impede the rehabilitation of a client with mental illness. Creating a list of issues about the client will help the worker establish a profile of the client. The worker can also derive treatment and action plans accordingly. Figure 3.2 illustrates this assessment framework.

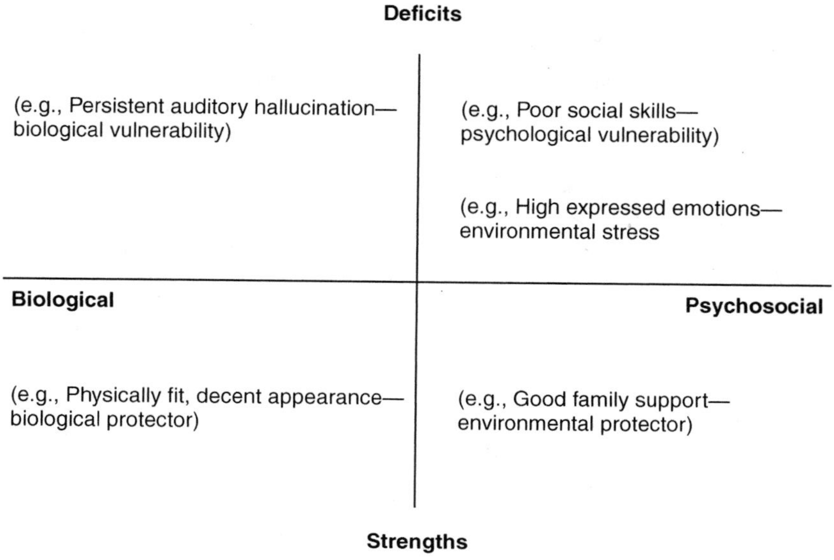

Deficits

(e.g., Persistent auditory hallucination—biological vulnerability)	(e.g., Poor social skills—psychological vulnerability)
	(e.g., High expressed emotions—environmental stress
Biological	**Psychosocial**
(e.g., Physically fit, decent appearance—biological protector)	(e.g., Good family support—environmental protector)

Strengths

FIGURE 3.2. Framework for a Biopsychosocial Vulnerability-Stress Model of Psychiatric Assessment

Medical/Physical Aspects

Generally speaking, the major focus of assessment in this medical and physical aspect includes: the understanding of a client's current mental state, a client's pattern of relapse, and the effects of the illness on a person's functioning. Specific areas of assessment in this aspect are presented in the following sections.

History of Psychiatric Illness

Onset of illness. It is important to know whether the illness is developed in a short period of time (acute onset) or has been developed over a relatively long period of time (insidious onset). If the onset is acute, the prognosis is usually better. On the other hand, if the onset is insidious, the prognosis may be poor. In fact, some clients may have developed symptoms (e.g., apathy or lack of volition) for so long that it is difficult to help them improve their situation. It is useful for family members and workers to have such knowledge because it helps them make realistic expectations of the client's rehabilitation progress.

Family history of psychiatric illness. It is not uncommon to find that a person with mental illness has other family members suffering from a similar type of mental illness as well. When more than one family member has the illness, the chance of the illness being genetically determined is greater (e.g., schizophrenia). Therefore, it is useful to ask the client whether any family member has a mental illness.

Numbers, circumstances, and reasons for admission to hospitals. It is necessary to understand the severity of the illness (e.g., involving self-harm or not), the symptoms manifestations (e.g., type of visual hallucination experienced by the client), and circumstances leading to hospitalization or relapse (e.g., specific environmental stressors, drug compliance, and ways in which the client copes with the situation). This information is extremely useful in preventing relapse. In clinical practice, it is not uncommon to find that a client usually manifests similar pattern of relapse. Knowing this can help the client and the worker identify early signs of relapse and develop strategies to deal with the issues before they become unmanageable.

Case example. Mrs. Tsui is fifty-eight years old, widowed, with a long history of schizophrenia. She lives on her own, and her son visits her once every two weeks. In one of our earlier counseling sessions she told me that whenever she felt "unwell" (starting to relapse) she could smell a certain unpleasant odor. She then believed that her neighbors were trying to poison her again. Subsequently, she would lock herself up and spray her house with a strong air freshener. She would yell at her neighbors and refuse to let anyone enter her house. It was discovered that Mrs. Tsui had stopped taking her medications a few months prior to her relapses. This information was very useful because I was able to identify her early signs of relapse. This successfully prevented her from having further psychotic relapses. In order to obtain such information, it is important to take a history of a client's relapse patterns in the beginning of the working relationship.

Attempts in coping with symptoms. What strategies did the client use previously to manage his or her symptoms, such as hallucinations, depressed moods, and anxiety states? How effective were these strategies? This information can help the worker to help the client develop alternative coping strategies to deal with his or her symptoms. This is often subsumed under the term *symptom management.*

Client understanding and acceptance of illness. This is known as *insight into illness.* Two reasons for tapping this information can be given. First, the client's understanding and acceptance of illness is closely related to his or her willingness to participate in the rehabilitation process. For example, it is quite common for clients who do not accept their mental illness to refuse to take their medications. Second, nonacceptance may lead to self-rejection or low self-esteem.

Coexistence of Physical and/or Psychiatric Illnesses

Primary or secondary diagnosis. A client may experience two types of illness and be medically treated with two types of drugs. However, clinically, the two illnesses may be distinguished as primary or secondary. For example, a person may have obsessive-compulsive disorder with depressed mood. In this case, depression is actually a result of the obsessive-compulsive disorder. Classifying the illnesses as primary or secondary helps to identify the major intervention focus. When the primary illness is successfully treated, the secondary illness will hopefully be lifted.

Other physical illnesses and medical conditions. Check whether the client has other illnesses. Other illnesses may complicate the treatment process. In fact, the worker needs to take the two illnesses into consideration when making a treatment plan. For example, in helping a client with intellectual disability to comply to his or her drug treatment regimen, complications may arise due to his or her limited intelligence.

However, more important, some symptoms of a certain mental illness may have an underlying physical/medical cause. It is necessary to identify and address this other cause rather than treat only the psychiatric symptoms. For example, a person with hypothyroidism may be diagnosed as having a depression because he or she exhibits depressive symptoms. Similarly, a young person with drug-induced psychosis may be diagnosed as having schizophrenia because of the presence of psychotic symptoms.

Medications

Type of medications being taken. It is important to know what types of medication the client is taking and the proper effects of these medications. This question *must* be asked during the interview. Mental health workers need to have some knowledge about psychotropic medications. Since workers are in close contact with clients, they can educate clients on the effects and side effects of the medications, inform medical staff of any adverse effects due to a change in medications, and negotiate with doctors regarding a reduction or an increase in medications due to the change in a client's mental state.

Side effects of medication. It is important to know the side effects of medication and discuss with the client the ways to managing these side effects. Some side effects are quite disturbing to the client, and he or she needs to know and be prepared for the side effects. Some clients may refuse to take lithium because it can lead to a loss of hair and weight gain. Other medications, such as the antipsychotics, can be very sedative and affect the daily functioning of the clients. Although it is necessary to try every means to help clients find ways of managing side effects, psychiatrists may need to be consulted regarding a change in the medication should the side effects be too severe for the clients.

Client's understanding and compliance to medications. It is always helpful to get a sense of whether the client will comply to medications. If he or she is not complying to the medications, he or she may have a greater chance of relapse. Therefore, the worker needs to explore the reasons why the client is not taking the medications and determine whether something can be done.

Alternative medicines. Some family members and clients in Hong Kong may take alternative Chinese medicines in addition to Western medicines. Although they cannot be denied their choices and decisions, they should be advised of any possible unhealthy side effects caused by mixing the two types of medicines together. Family members and clients are often willing to discuss this issue and can be encouraged to seek further advice from their psychiatrists.

Current Mental State (Mental State Examination)

A few points must be kept in mind when examining a client's current mental state. First, mental state examination focuses mainly on assessing the behaviors and the verbal and nonverbal contents of the client's utterances. Second, the worker needs to carefully observe as well as obtain a verbal report from the client. The worker must be cognizant of any discrepancy between the verbal and nonverbal expressions of the client. Third, the worker must look for subtle changes in the client's mental state. For example, one of my clients experienced residual auditory hallucinations of a woman's voice calling him a "bad boy." As the illness progressed, the frequency of the voice increased and the content of the voice changed and encouraged him to commit suicide. He would then become more distressed and agitated. These symptoms indicated that the client was starting to relapse. This example supports the need for the worker to take note of the subtle changes in the client's mental state and to periodically compare the client's current mental state to that of the previous weeks.

Many instruments facilitate a mental state examination (e.g., Lukoff, Nuechterlein, & Ventura, 1986). The following items are commonly included in a mental state examination:

1. Appearance—physical presentation, facial expressions, dress (e.g., unkempt appearance in cases of depression)
2. Motor activity—increased, decreased, or catatonic (e.g., reduced level of activities in the case of depression)
3. Mood and affect—emotional expressions in terms of range, changeability, or liability and appropriateness of affect (e.g., sudden mood swings in the case of manic depression)
4. Speech and language—latency of response, paucity of response, pressurized speech (e.g., poverty of speech in a person with schizophrenia)
5. Thought content—ruminating thoughts, obsessive thoughts, phobic thoughts, delusional thoughts (e.g., recurrent thought of being persecuted by neighbors)
6. Perceptual disturbances—hallucinations, depersonalization, and derealization (e.g., constantly experiencing auditory hallucination)
7. Insight and judgment—insight into illness and ability to make correct decisions
8. Neuropsychiatric functions—level of consciousness, attention and concentration, memory and orientation to time, place and object (e.g., a demented elderly with poor memory and loss of orientation to time, place, and objects)

It is worth noting that a combination of symptoms gathered from an examination of the previously outlined areas may give an impression of the type of illness a client may be having. For example, a client is likely to be experiencing a manic state if he or she has elevated moods, increased motor activities, an unkempt appearance, pressurized speech, excessive energy level, and/or participates in reckless activities. Although it is the responsibility of the psychiatrist to make a clinical diagnosis of the client, it is important for mental health workers to systematically examine the client and provide the psychiatrist with the current information on his or her mental state. This information is essential for successful monitoring of the rehabilitation process of the client.

Social and Family Aspects

These aspects of assessment focus on two major areas: identifying the functional skills essential for an individual to enact desired social, occupational, and instrumental roles; and assessing the resources and constraints that exist in an individual's social and family relationships and identifying the stress and vulnerability factors.

Social Aspect

Skills for social role performance. This set of skills can be generally subsumed under social skills. Although these skills may be referred to as verbal and nonverbal communication skills (e.g., Trower et al., 1986), they can also be defined as the specific skills needed to fulfill a specific social role. It is assumed that the inability to perform adequately in these social roles can create great stress for clients. For example, a client needs to learn specific skills when he becomes a father. A mental health worker should assess whether a client is capable of performing basic communication skills and other skills necessary for performing certain social roles (Appendix I).

Skills for independent living. This is another set of skills that many clients with chronic mental illness must learn in order to live independently in a community. These skills include self-care skills, domestic-living skills, health-maintenance skills, community-living skills, and money-management skills. It is not uncommon for workers to use a checklist approach to assess a client's overall level of skill performance in the different skill areas.

Other social and environmental conditions. It is essential to examine the social and environmental conditions that may constitute resources or stresses to the client. These environments may include a client's school, living conditions, social network, and job situation. Each environment can either be a curative or a stress factor for the client. If an environment is not conducive to the rehabilitation of the client, the worker must either help the client learn to adapt to the environment or to remove him or her from the environment. Moreover, the worker may have to identify and link the client to suitable community resources.

Family Aspect

Composition, nature of relationships. It is helpful to get a profile of the client's family composition and identify the members who are supportive and unsupportive. Since family members, particularly the caregiver, have the most contact with the client, they can provide current information about the mental state of the client.

Possible impact of the illness on family members. Much attention is put toward helping the client with the illness, and family members quite often become the silent victims who must bear tremendous burdens in taking care of their loved ones with chronic mental illness. Many studies have found that family members experience much stress and mental ill health when caring for the relative with a chronic mental illness (e.g., Wong, 2000). Excessive stress can affect the quality of relationships between the family members and the client, leading to conflict and rejection. An intense family atmosphere characterized by critical comments, overinvolvement, and hostility is associated with a higher rate of relapse. It is important to identify these stress factors in the family.

Family attitudes toward illness and interventions. Family members sometimes have different perceptions of the cause of illness and of the type of treatment that is best for their relative. It is important to understand their views so that their attitudes do not become obstacles that block the treatment process. For example, family members of one of my clients strongly believed that Western medicines were harmful to his brother's body and could not cure the disease. They deliberately discouraged the brother from taking the medications and took him to China to receive many different traditional herbal treatments and to participate in ritualistic practices. These various forms of treatment proved unsuccessful, and in some instances cause harmful side effects for the client. Consequently, the situation was discussed with the family members and a compromise was reached.

Attempts of the family members to cope with illness. Each family may have developed a unique pattern of relating to and handling their relative with mental illness. Some family members may make the mentally ill relative a scapegoat for other family problems. Others may see themselves as responsible for causing the illness, and react with undue sacrifice. Through family interviews, the caseworker can get a sense of how family members perceive and cope with the illness. In some cases, it is more helpful to adopt a family approach to treatment.

Case example. Harry was diagnosed as having a "personality problem" and had been physically abusive toward his wife and daughters for the past few years. He was discharged to our halfway house for further rehabilitation. Although he wanted to return home as soon as possible, other family members strongly rejected the idea. Upon further probing, it was found that his daughters and his wife were very afraid of him because his violent behaviors were unpredictable. Their usual pattern of response was to withdraw and distance themselves emotionally and physically. Individual interviews with Harry revealed that he felt very lonely and useless, largely because he was retired and had to rely on his daughters for financial support. He did not have many friends, did not enjoy social activities, and had not developed any hobbies. This was a family in which members were not used to communicating feelings and support. A family approach to treatment was used and family members were encouraged to express their feelings to one another, helping them understand one another in a way they had not done before.

Vocational Aspects

Vocational assessment should provide the worker the following information about his or her client: impact of the illness on the vocational functioning of a client, personal and interpersonal factors that affect the client's occupational functioning, the training potential of the client, and the resources needed to support the client.

Present Job Situations

If the person has a job, it is useful to find out information such as the nature of the job, relationships with colleagues, satisfaction with the job, and the effects of illness on the client's job performance. This information can help the worker identify any stress factors that may affect the mental state of the client, and can also help the worker evaluate the impact of psychiatric impairments on the job performance of the client.

Past Work History and Performance

The worker needs to take a detailed history of a client's past work record. By doing this the worker is able to understand the circumstances and factors related to illness, personality, and environmental constraints on the client's work ability and performance. Moreover, a client's ways of coping with the problems at work can also be revealed. This information can facilitate the planning of prevocational and vocational training and of vocational counseling for the client.

Prevocational Skills

Clients with chronic mental illness may need to undergo prevocational skills assessment in order to understand whether they have the basic work skills necessary for future employment. Occupational therapists have the expertise and the equipment to conduct this assessment. In Hong Kong, occupational therapy departments within hospitals provide prevocational assessment for the clients.

Vocational Interests and Skills

Some clients may need vocational skills training before they can take on a new job. The worker should discuss vocational interests with the client and identify ways he or she can turn these interests into vocational goals. The worker should also link the client to training sites and resources that will help him or her learn the necessary skills needed for the desired job. Currently in Hong Kong sheltered employment and supported employment aim to provide vocational skills training for persons with mental illness.

Psychological Aspects

Identifying Cognitive Dysfunctions

As discussed in Chapter 2, cognition plays a vital role in determining an individual's emotional outcomes. Indeed, human behaviors and problems are directly related to how a person responds to the world. Three cognitive elements are involved in the functional processes: (1) automatic thoughts, (2) intermediate beliefs, and (3) core beliefs (Beck, 1995). *Automatic thoughts* refer to reflexive self-statements or images that an individual involuntarily experiences throughout daily life. An individual experiencing negative automatic thoughts misinterprets a situation and negatively distorts its reality. This distorted interpretation is heavily influenced by the person's schema, which includes both intermediate beliefs and core beliefs. *Intermediate beliefs* are rules, assumptions, and attitudes a person holds, and *core beliefs* are underlying, unconscious, rigidly held beliefs that influence both intermediate beliefs and automatic thoughts. For example, if a person appraises himself or herself as inadequate, he or she may hold such rules and assumptions (intermediate thoughts) as "Whatever I have accomplished is because someone else has made it possible" and "No matter how hard I try, I can never make it." An individual having intermediate beliefs may experience different types of cognitive distortions (automatic thoughts), interpreting specific events incorrectly. If an employer comments negatively on the individual's performance on a certain task, he or she may remark, "I have made a complete mess of the situation," even if he or she has made only a small mistake, the task was otherwise completed smoothly and on time (selective abstraction). Finally, these cognitive processes affect how a person behaves and feels. Using the previous example, since the employee thinks he or she has made a mess of the situation, the individual feels very disappointed and shameful and avoids making contact with colleagues and bosses. In the assessment process, the worker needs to be aware of the client's cognitive processes and how they influence the client's behaviors and emotions. Simply put, these cognitive processes put the person in a vulnerable position for developing mental illness during stressful circumstances.

Identifying and Facilitating the Expression of Emotions

Emotion is an integral part of a person's personality. It affects and is affected by one's thoughts, behavior, and physiology. Negative, excessive, restricted, or inappropriate emotions are as signs and symptoms of different types of mental health problems. For example, whereas depression is characterized by excessively low moods and negative emotions such as guilt and self-blame, anxiety problems are expressed through excessive worries and fear. Different processes may be involved in creating the emotional problems experienced by an individual. These processes include denying and suppressing one's inner yearning and yielding to others' demands, inability to fulfill one's goals and aspirations, and traumatic experiences in life. In the assessment process, it is important to identify (1) how well the person is in expressing his or her emotions—are they appropriate, restricted, or excessive? and (2) the underlying factors that influence the expression of emotions. To achieve this, the worker should help the individual express and experience his or her emotions and become aware of how his or her emotions may have contributed to his or her emotional disturbances; should create a therapeutic relationship in which the client can explore his or her own interests, goals, and aspirations; and should find ways to fulfilling these goals.

Identifying Low Self-Esteem in Clients

It is not uncommon to find that some people with mental illness have low self-esteem. Although this may have been a result of a long-standing experience of personal failure, some may have developed a low self-esteem as a consequence of his or her illness. Some clients have found themselves unable to do what they used to do and have come to accept a low quality of life characterized by such factors as a poorly paying job and poor housing conditions. People with mental illness are alienated from participating in social and occupational activities. This social and self-stigma can further hamper self-esteem. Consequently, such low self-esteem may affect the motivation of some illness suffers to actively participate in the rehabilitation process. Therefore, the worker needs to assess the client's self-esteem level and how it be affecting the client's rehabilitation.

MICROSKILLS IN ASSESSMENT

Active Listening

Worker should be constantly aware of the nonverbal and verbal expression of the clients. Workers should listen carefully to clients' expressions with the objective of understanding their experiences of joys, sadness, pain, endurance, etc. When workers are willing to do this, their clients should then be able to establish a trustful and respectful relationship. Assessment is the workers' attempts to reach out and try to understand their clients' total experiences. Sometimes workers may not be able to fully understand the clients' expressions (e.g., hallucinations). However, workers' genuine interest and concern will keep the relationship going in a meaningful direction.

Balancing Information Gathering and Attending to Client's Physical and Emotional States

During the assessment process it is easy for the worker to make the mistake of becoming too involved in getting information and ignoring the emotional state of the client. It is important for the worker to be aware of the client's emotional state and to show support during the interview. It is advisable to let the client say as much as he or she is able and willing to say, and not to push beyond his or her limit. In a trustful and comfortable relationship, a client is more willing to disclose himself or herself to the worker. Basic interviewing skills such as reflection of content and reflection of feelings are quite useful in these circumstances.

Don't Argue with the Client About His or Her Delusion or Hallucination

It is unhelpful to argue with the client about his or her delusion or hallucination, particularly during the assessment phase. The more the worker argues with the client on such issues, the more defensive the client becomes. Moreover, the client would be less likely to establish a trustful relationship with the worker. It would be helpful for the worker to focus on and respond to the client's feeling that is attached to the delusion and hallucination (e.g., "You seem to be very unhappy about hearing this voice"). The worker is not showing agreement to the client's delusion or hallucination; the worker is conveying his or her understanding of the client's difficulties and concerns.

When Family Members Are Present in the Assessment Interview

Even if family members are present, workers should remember that their principal concern is still the client. Therefore, questions should be asked directly to the client as much as possible. It is not uncommon to have a dominant family member jump in to express his or her views when a question is asked, or to have a family member express strong emotion during the interview. In these circumstances a balance should be struck, and a space for the client to talk should always be provided. Moreover, occasions will occur when the worker will need to gently remind the family member to give the client room to express himself or herself.

CASE ILLUSTRATION

Background

Janet is a thirty-six-year-old divorced woman suffering from schizophrenia. Her first known psychiatric episode took place nine years previously. The community psychiatric treatment (CPT) team visited Janet after receiving complaints from neighbors that she placed feces on their doorsteps. When the police inspected her apartment, they found it full of garbage and totally unhygienic. She was then sent to a nearby hospital for further psychiatric assessment. Eventually, she was admitted to a major psychiatric hospital and remained in the hospital for three years.

Medical/Physical Aspects

It was found that prior to admission Janet had at least a one-year history of abnormal behaviors and beliefs. According to the police record, she had made several complaints about her neighbors, saying that they had broken into her apartment and had stolen from her. She became so insecure and angry at the neighbors that she decided to take revenge by putting feces on their doorsteps. She also maintained that the police were unhelpful and could not stop her neighbors from stealing from her. She was unswerving about this belief. In the hospital, she complained about other patients and acted aggressively toward one of them. She was eventually given a hospital order and was sent to another hospital. Upon the completion of her sentence, she was sent back to the first hospital for further treatment.

At home, she was unkempt and had very poor hygiene. She seldom took baths or washed her clothes. She explained, "I do not sweat easily. There is no need to take a bath. I'll do it when I have sweated." She did not realize that she smelled bad and that she had developed skin problems. The nursing staff had difficulty supervising her self-care, and she reacted angrily toward them. On a few occasions she was rather aggressive.

Since admission, she had been put on antipsychotic medications. Although she experienced some side effects, such as dry mouth and constipation, she was rather settled and calm. She spoke coherently and relevantly. She did not report any hallucinations and did not experience any cognitive dysfunctions. However, she harbored residual delusions against her neighbors, but with less anger and frustration. Further probing suggested that Janet had not developed a more adaptive coping strategy to handle her delusion. As she claimed, "If I spot them stealing things from me again, I am going to call the police. If they can't help, I'll call the mayor. They must be stopped." Indeed, Janet had very poor insight into her illness and refused to see this delusion as part of her illness manifestations. When asked why she was willing to take the medication, she replied: "The doctor said it is good for me, so I take it. But it doesn't make any difference to me."

Family and Social Aspects

Janet has six siblings. She is the fifth sibling in the family. Both parents died a few years ago. None of the family members has any history of mental illness. One of Janet's older sisters is supportive of her and visits her monthly. This sister took care of Janet's five-year-old child while she was in the hospital. However, Janet had never taken care of her daughter since her birth and had no knowledge of any child care skills and facilities. She said, "I don't expect any problems. My child will grow naturally as we did. We had no problem in the past." Janet was very eager to live with her daughter and was adamant that she could take good care of her. She also maintained that her sister would lend her a helping hand should she need any assistance.

Janet used to live in a public housing estate, and would be granted an apartment when she returned to the community. She said she had lived in the community independently for many years and did not foresee any problem. Although she did not seem to have adequate self-care, domestic-living, or health-maintenance skills, she did not see any need to acquire these skills. However, she said she preferred to live close to her older sister because her sister could help her when needed.

Socially, Janet has only a few acquaintances. She said, "I don't know where my friends are. I have lost contact with them for years. Well, I know a few patients who used to live in this hospital. Maybe I can call them when I get out of the hospital." By and large, she has a rather small network of acquaintances and family members.

Vocational Aspects

Janet had worked as a salesgirl and a factory worker. Neither job lasted for more than six months. She does not know why she cannot hold a job for a longer period of time, but blames bosses and colleagues for mistreating her. She says she did not speak very much with others and felt that her colleagues did not like her and acted together against her. Eventually she stopped working and relied on welfare assistance for four years prior to admission. In one of the interviews, Janet claimed that she could find and maintain a job if she wanted to. She also mentioned that one of the ex-patients of the hospital promised to get her a job as a cleaner if discharged. She said, "It is easy to be a cleaner. Everyone knows how to clean a place."

Psychological Aspect

Janet has developed a distorted view about other's intentions to mistreat her. These delusional experiences might be partly related to her illness and partly reinforced by her life experiences. Regardless of her mental stability she continues to harbor delusions regarding her neighbors and others. Janet also has problems with impulse control. When angry or unhappy she unleashes her emotions without considering the circumstances or consequences. In her words, "This is always a part of me. I don't like people bossing me around." This attitude had brought about many interpersonal conflicts between Janet and others in the past. As a consequence, Janet mentioned that she withdrew and preferred to live alone.

Overall Assessment

Although Janet continued to harbor delusions about her neighbors, she could be considered mentally stable. First, she did not act on her delusions. Second, her delusions did not seem to be affecting her social and occupational functioning. Third, she did not manifest other major signs and symptoms of schizophrenia and spoke coherently and relevantly. Finally, she was compliant with medications and took them regularly in the hospital. However, compliance might be a cause of concern when she returned to the community, because without supervision Janet might not take the medications (deficit—lacking a biological protector). Without medications she might lose control of and act on her delusions. Janet could benefit from a better understanding of her mental illness and of the effects and side effects of her medications. She should also learn some adaptive coping strategies to handle her delusions (deficit—personal vulnerability factor). It might not be possible for Janet to ever be rid of her delusions, but she could respond differently to her delusions.

Socially, Janet had poor independent-living skills and child care skills (deficit—psychological vulnerability factor). Although it was debatable whether Janet should be encouraged to pursue her choice of living, it would be totally unacceptable for the child to live with a mother who could not even take care of herself. Should Janet prefer to live with her child in the future (deficit—environmental stress factor), the worker would need to help her to develop independent-living skills and self-care skills. This would be a great challenge to both

Janet and the worker. However, this could be a possible motivational factor for Janet to make some changes in her life (strength—psychological protector). Moreover, Janet has an older sister who is very supportive of her, and this network should further be strengthened (strength—environmental protector). She might also benefit a great deal from developing some supportive relationships with others (this would depend on the severity of her delusions in the future).

Psychologically, several factors might affect Janet's rehabilitation. Although her delusions could be considered a biological factor relating to her psychiatric illness, these delusions had obviously affected and would affect her perception and judgment in the future (deficit—psychological vulnerability factor). Due to incorrect perceptions, Janet got into arguments and conflicts with others easily. Moreover, Janet had impulse-control problems and would act and react impulsively (deficit—psychological vulnerability factor). This seriously affected her relationships with others, leading to adverse social, vocational, and could even lead to legal consequences.

Several factors might affect Janet's future job situation. First, although Janet claimed she could secure a job, her past job records were not very positive. Indeed, she might benefit from further job assessment before the worker helps Janet made any concrete plan for future employment (deficit—psychological stress factor). Second, if Janet lived with her daughter, it would affect whether she could work or not as well as the type of employment she could have. Nonetheless, some kinds of job assessment might still be called for.

In general, Janet would benefit from living in a supervised facility such as a halfway house for a certain period of time before living on her own. During the period, Janet could be facilitated in acquiring better drug compliance, developing adequate independent living and child care skills, and she could undergo prevocational and vocational assessment.

As the biopsychosocial vulnerability-stress model of psychiatric assessment shows, it is essential for a mental health worker to identify the various biological and psychosocial factors influencing the mental health of an individual and to evaluate whether these factors are vulnerability and environmental stress factors or biological and environmental protectors. This proposed model appreciates both the deficits incurred in having a mental illness as well as the strengths an individual has and can develop during the recovery process.

Chapter 4

Depression

INTRODUCTION

Depression (major depressive disorder) is a type of mood disorder in DSM-IV-TR classification. It is a very common mental illness in Hong Kong, and about one-quarter of the total population experience depression at least once in their lifetime. According to the *Rehabilitation Programme Plan Review* (Health and Welfare Bureau, 1999), only 10 percent of the people suffering from major depression will require psychiatric rehabilitation services. Many are treated by private psychiatrists, general practitioners, counselors, and social workers belonging to nongovernment organizations. Twice the number of females develop depression compared to males. Besides major depressive disorder, other mood disorders are dysthymic disorder (a prolonged minor depression of at least two years exhibiting symptoms of depression not warranting a diagnosis of major depression), and cyclothymic disorder (numerous episodes of hypomania and minor depression but not warranting a diagnosis of bipolar disorder) (American Psychiatric Association, 2000). This chapter focuses on delineating assessments and interventions for people suffering from major depressive disorder, because the most commonly diagnosed mood disorder is major depression. The principles and skills of working with persons with major depression can often be applied to dysthymic disorder, however, these principles and skills may not be useful for helping people in the manic phase of manic depression or for those with cyclothymic disorder.

ASSESSING A PERSON WITH DEPRESSION

Four areas must be assessed: (1) medical and biological aspects, (2) emotional aspects, (3) cognitive aspects, and (4) interpersonal and family aspects.

Medical and Biological Aspects

History of Depression

It is important to understand whether the person or a member of his or her other family has a history of depression. People with family members who are suffering from or have had depression have a higher prevalence rate of depression that those without a family history. Likewise, the chance of a recurrent depression is also higher among those who have a previous history of depression (Gotlib & Colby, 1987). Understanding the person's history of depression is useful for distinguishing whether he or she has an endogenous or a reactive depression. In the case of *endogenous depression,* the person is more likely to be genetically predisposed to the illness. In biomedical terms, the person has an irregularly low level of serotonin and/or an irregularly low level of norepinephrine (both are neurotransmitters) in the brain (Diziegielewski & Leon, 1998). Therefore, he or she needs medication to restore biochemical balance in the brain. However, some individuals with endogenous depression may not be responsive to antidepressants and can experience numerous bouts of depression during his or her lifetime. Although they are still likely to be put on antidepressants, such sufferers need ongoing supportive counseling from mental health workers. The focus of counseling for those with endogenous depression is to help them adjust to a chronic depressive condition so that they can maintain optimum functioning in society. On the other hand, *reactive depression* is related to interpersonal and environmental factors such as stress, death of a family member, unemployment, separation, etc. (Gotlib & Colby, 1987). Reactive depression is more amendable to counseling than is endogenous. It is believed that when the interpersonal and environmental problems causing depression are resolved, these individuals are likely to recover completely from depression. However, in some cases they may initially be put on antidepressants along with undergoing counseling. The mental health worker should periodically assess clients' changes in mood and discuss with psychiatrists the possibility of reducing and even ceasing the antidepressants prescribed to the clients.

Treatment Received and Coping Methods Used

The mental health worker must explore the types of treatment received by the person before and during hospitalization, the stressors that lead to depression, and the client's previous coping strategies used to deal with the symptoms of depression. It is useful for the worker to know the types of medications and other medical treatments that the client received in the past and how he or she responded to the treatments. It is worthwhile to explore whether the client had taken or is taking any alternative medicines such as Chinese herbal medicines. When exploring the client's history of hospitalization, it is useful to examine the type of stressors that lead to the recurrence of depression. The worker should look for a similar pattern of stressors. If this pattern is identified, the worker can help the client develop strategies to deal with the stressors. The key point is to look for a pattern. For example, one client of mine became depressed rather frequently because she could not cope with difficulties in interpersonal relationships. She would often withdraw from relationships and engage in very negative, self-deprecating thoughts. We then discussed thoroughly her pattern of responses to difficulties in interpersonal relationships. As she began to realize her pattern of responses she was able to avoid as well as develop coping skills to handle the stressful interpersonal relationships. Finally, the worker needs to know how the client is managing his or her symptoms of depression. For example, a client is lethargic and spends much time at home and does not participate in any social activities. He tends to ruminate about lost relationship. The worker should recognize that this behavior perpetuates the client's symptoms of withdrawal. Thus, it is important to understand a client's maladaptive coping methods and to help him or her develop alternate and adaptive methods.

Secondary Depression

For treatment purposes, it is necessary to distinguish between primary and secondary depression. Secondary depression can be a symptom of another, primary mental illness. For example, a person diagnosed with schizophrenia may present depressive symptoms generated from his or her fear that he or she is being persecuted by others. Another instance of secondary depression can occur in a person with obsessive-compulsive disorder (OCD). Since he or she cannot deal with the intrusive thoughts and the compulsive acts, he or she becomes depressed. In these circumstances the primary illnesses are schizophrenia and obsessive-compulsive disorder. Depression is secondary to these illnesses. Although antidepressants are often helpful for individuals with secondary depression, the treatment focus should center on the primary illnesses. It is worth mentioning that some physical illnesses may also cause depression-like symptoms. It is important to rule out these possible causes before making a diagnosis that the person has primary depression. For example, a person with hypothyroidism often experiences depressive symptoms, and it is disadvantageous for the person to acquire a socially stigmatizing label of mental illness and is counterproductive to treatment.

Severity of Depression

The severity of depression is determined by (1) duration of symptoms/illness, (2) impact of the illness on the social and occupational functioning, and (3) insight into illness and compliance with medications.

Duration of symptoms/illness. A person who is diagnosed as having major depressive disorder must satisfy the DSM-IV-TR criteria with either a depressed mood or loss of interest in once-pleasurable activities along with four other symptoms of depression (for example, change in sleep patterns or appetite, increased fatigue, feelings of guilt, and others outlined in the DSM-IV-TR). Second, these symptoms must be present for at least two weeks in order to be diagnosed as clinical depression. In practice, it is useful to ask the client pointed questions such as the following in order to differentiate whether the person is clinically depressed. For example, "In the past two weeks, has your appetite changed?" and "In the past two weeks, have you had any obvious weight gain or loss? How much have you gained or lost?" However, during interviews, it may not be appropriate to use a checklist approach to tap the client's symptoms. Rather, it is more natural to let the client express his or her concerns and ask questions at appropriate moments. For example, if a client mentions how much he or she misses his or her son after a divorce and how unhappy it has made him or her, the worker might then ask "Besides feeling unhappy, how does this affect your sleep and appetite?"

Impact on social and occupational functioning. If the person manifests symptoms of depression that do not significantly affect his or her functioning (e.g., work), he or she is not considered to have severe depression. Those who are clinically depressed are usually unable to perform some or most of the social and occupational roles that he or she can normally do.

Case example: Susan lost her husband and a son in the same year. She exhibits symptoms of depression including extremely low mood, loss of interest in formerly enjoyable activites, substantial weight loss, poor appetite, crying, and feelings of worthlessness. These symptoms lasted for more than a month. Her other son who lived apart took notice of his mother's changing conditions and contacted our community health center for help. Her son told us that her house was a mess and his mother looked disheveled. The refrigerator was empty, and it seemed as though she had not cooked food in a while. In the past, his mother was a diligent housewife who would not tolerate an untidy and tainted house. In this case, depression had affected the mother's normal functioning.

Insight into illness and compliance to medications. People with depression do not normally lose insight about their illnesses. However, some clients perceive their depressive symptoms differently and do not want to seek treatment or comply with medications. It is important for the worker to explore their clients' views and help them to come to grips with their depression. For example, a client of mine refused to take medication even though she had severe symptoms of depression. She could entertain only the idea that she could not sleep and eat properly because she had marital conflicts with her husband. It took her a while before she could accept that she might be clinically depressed and need medication.

In addition to hospitalization, another question that a mental health worker needs to ask is: Does the person need psychotropic medications or is counseling a better option? The worker has to examine each option carefully. Medication should be considered for those clients who have endogenous depression or who have severe reactive depression that is seriously affecting their functioning. In many of these cases, both medications and counseling are needed. Whereas medications stabilize the moods of those with severe depression, counseling can help these individuals work through the issues troubling them or to learn skills to manage their depressive symptoms. The mental health worker also provides intensive counseling for those who are depressed but do not require medication. However, should the mental health worker suspect that the client needs medication, he or she should refer the client for psychiatric assessment.

Medical Treatments

Hospitalization. An examination of the severity of depression should help the worker decide whether a client should be hospitalized. Generally speaking, a client with symptoms of clinical depression can be a suitable candidate for hospitalization. However, two other factors are often taken into consideration: whether the person has any suicidal thoughts or plans and/or whether he or she has someone who supports him or her in the community. If the person is clinically depressed, has a suicidal plan, and does not have a good support network in the community, the worker should recommend hospitalization for this person.

Drug treatment. It is suggested that antidepressants are particularly effective for people with severe depression. Several types of antidepressants are used for treating depressive disorders. These include the SSRIs (selective serotonin reuptake inhibitors) (e.g., Prozac and Luvox), tricyclic antidepressants (TCAs) (e.g., Toframil and Nopramin), and the monoamine oxidase inhibitors (MAOIs) (e.g., Nardil and Parnate) (Diziegielewski & Leon, 1998). The SSRIs generally have fewer side effects than tricyclics. Although some improvements may be seen in the first few weeks, antidepressant medications must be taken regularly for at least three to four weeks before the full therapeutic effect occurs. It is important to keep taking medication until it has a chance to work, though the side effects may appear before the antidepressant takes effect. Once the individual is feeling better, it is important to continue the medication for at least four to nine months to prevent a recurrence of the depression.

Antidepressants may cause mild and, usually, temporary side effects (sometimes referred to as adverse effects). The most common side effects of TCAs are dry month, constipation, bladder problems, and sexual problems. The SSRIs have different types of side effects: headache, nausea, nervousness and insomnia, and sexual problems.

In any case, if the client complains about any of these problems, the mental health worker should instruct him or her to consult a doctor.

Electroconvulsive therapy. ECT may be administered to people with severe depression who do not responded well to antidepressants (Diziegielewski & Leon, 1998). In recent years, ECT has been much improved. A muscle relaxant is given before treatment, which is done under brief anesthesia. Electrodes are placed at precise locations on the head to deliver electrical impulses. The stimulation causes a brief (about thirty seconds) seizure within the brain. The person receiving ECT does not consciously experience the electrical stimulus. For full therapeutic benefit, at least several sessions of ECT, typically given at the rate of three per week, are required.

Roles of Mental Health Workers in Addressing the Medical Needs of a Depressed Client

Clients may not have much knowledge of depression. One of the worker's roles is to educate the client about depression, and about the medications and their side effects. It is believed that the more clients understand the issues involved, the better they are able to accept their illness and comply with medical treatment.

Another role of the mental health worker is to monitor a client's mental state and medication closely. It is important for the worker to take note of the client's subtle changes in mood and other symptoms, in both positive and negative directions. This information can be given to the client's doctor for medical management, and it can also be used to facilitate therapeutic changes in a client. When a client expresses a subtle improvement in his or her mood, the worker can capitalize on the change by inviting the client to give further details as to what he or she has done that makes the change possible. This technique is quite useful for a client with depression because he or she tends to overlook the positives and focus on the negatives (Beck, Rush, Shaw, & Emery, 1979), thus continuously trapped in his or her depression.

Emotional Aspects

Three points about the emotional aspect of depression deserve attention. These are: (1) depressed mood, (2) opportunity to express emotion, and (3) interventions focused on affective components.

Depressed Mood

Emotions can overshadow the life of a client. When the person is severely depressed, his or her depressed mood can seriously affect his or her daily functioning. He or she cannot sleep at night and does not have the motivation to perform tasks essential for social and occupational functioning. Indeed, he or she seems to have lost interest in doing anything, and does not have the energy to break through the depressed mood. This depressed mood forms part of a vicious cycle that puts the person into a prolonged and more severe depression. Essentially, the severely depressed client is in a state of low mood, withdraws from other people, does not interact with others, and is unable to get support and positive feedback or reinforcement from others. This may reinforce his or her negative thought that "no one cares." Subsequently, it further lowers his or her mood and the vicious cycle continues. This is portrayed graphically in Figure 4.1.

Therefore, changing a client's mood state becomes an important initial intervention point for helping him or her to get out of depression. Clinical experiences show that if the person's mood state is very low, it is unlikely that he or she can engage in any counseling work. The client's depressed mood has become so overbearing that he or she is symbolically "tied" to the mood state. The person needs a great

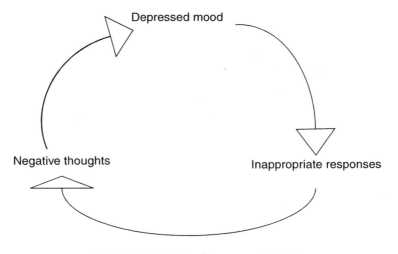

FIGURE 4.1. Cycle of Depressed Moods

amount of energy to break through this mood barrier. Indeed, unless the person's mood state is sufficiently uplifted, he or she may not have the energy to engage in any other intervention strategies.

Opportunity to Express Emotion

Clients with reactive depression encounter at least one major negative life event preceding the episode. These events may include losses, traumas, and sudden unexpected life events, causing an array of negative emotions. Clinical experiences have shown that these individuals need much time and opportunity to fully release emotions such as grief and loss, shock, and pain. Unless they can release these emotions, they may not be able to work on these issues actively and positively. On the other hand, although it is helpful for the clients to repeatedly talk about their issues during the initial period of counseling, it is unhealthy for them to continue to talk about their issues with the same frequency and intensity. Indeed, when the counseling sessions are therapeutic and the clients are gradually recovering from their depression, they should be able to talk about such subjects with less frequency and fewer negative emotions. Moreover, nonverbally, these clients have more positive features such as smiling, eye contact, quicker response time, and more energy. It is important for the worker to take notice of the positive changes and point them out to their clients. This encourages clients to feel that they are making some changes in their conditions.

Interventions Focused on Affective Components

Help the client to fully express his or her feelings. The worker should create a therapeutic environment in which the client feels safe to express his or her feelings and views about the negative life events. Once he or she is able to let out their feelings, the chance of falling further into the vicious cycle of depressed mood can be greatly reduced. The worker must give the client sufficient support so that he or she feels safe to express themselves. Some useful skills subsumed under the person-centered therapy are: unconditional positive regard, empathy, and congruence.

Help the client to work through issues regarding loss, grief, and other experiences. The worker should gently encourage the client to express such emotion such as grief and loss, should listen carefully to the client's concerns, should make adequate and appropriate reflections, and should avoid making judgments. Moreover, it is important to allow the client as much time as he or she needs, and, above all, to accept silence. Do not expect a client to speak when he or she is unable to. In this circumstance, the worker should show his or her understanding toward the client's difficulty to express himself or herself, and tell the client that it is all right to stay that way. It is also unhelpful if the worker, knowingly or unknowingly, avoids the "sensitive topics." Times will occur when a client has difficulty talking about some painful, unhappy, and embarrassing issues. The worker should not impulsively dig into the client's issues, instead, he or she needs to help the client gradually talk about these issues. For example, a severely depressed client may harbor thoughts of committing suicide. In the interview, he or she may have difficulty expressing this thought but also may feel very frustrated and fearful about not being able to control suicidal impulses. The worker should be aware of such difficulties and invite the client to express these thoughts.

Help the client monitor and change his or her emotions. Since the client will tend to dwell on the negatives, it is therapeutic for the worker to gradually encourage him or her to explore the positive changes in emotions and behaviors. When the worker notices any slight but positive changes in client's emotions and behaviors, the worker should encourage the client to examine these changes and capitalize on the efforts that have brought the changes about. In addition to observation and reflection, the worker can also use a scaling technique to help the client to talk about the change in his or her emotions. For example, a client is asked to rate on a scale of 1 to 10 (with 1 being unhappy, low mood and 10 being happy, very good mood) his or her state of emotion in the past week. The worker can then compare the current score with the previous week's score. If a difference occurs between the two scores, the client should be encouraged to explain the reasons that caused the difference. This is a useful technique because it helps the client keep track of his or her feelings and explore the circumstances leading to such feelings.

Cognitive Aspects

Beck et al. (1979) suggest that a depressed person has developed a cognitive triad in seeing the world, future, and the self negatively. The person may see oneself as worthless, the world as being cold and unfriendly, and the future as gloomy. Indeed, this person has acquired a sense of hopelessness. According to Beck, two cognitive processing issues are directly related to the formation of cognitive triad and hopelessness in a client. These are: (1) depressive schemata (core beliefs and intermediate beliefs, see Chapters 2 and 3) and (2) cognitive distortions (negative automatic thoughts, see Chapters 2 and 3). Interventions should be cognitively focused.

Depressive Schemata

Depressive schemata are cognitive structures that affect the information processing of a depressed person. In other words, the person develops certain rules for and beliefs about himself or herself and others, and since these rules and beliefs are transformed into expectations and interpretative references, they affect how the person interprets the intentions and actions of another person and how he or she subsequently responds to this person. Gilbert (2000) identified five types of depressive schemata, and claimed that these schemata are present in people with depression.

> *Approval schema:* "I am nothing or empty without love."
> *Achievement schema:* "I must succeed and be recognized."
> *Self-worth schema:* "I have nothing of value to contribute to others."
> *Efficacy schema:* "I can do nothing to change the situation."
> *Power schema:* "Others are more capable than I."

Individuals who rigidly adhere to any one of these schemata are vulnerable to becoming unhappy. For example, a mother with strong achievement schema will view her daughter's success or failure in school as an indication of her achievement or failure. If her daughter does not do well in school, she will be unhappy with her daughter and herself. This achievement schema will also affect the woman's perceptions of and expectation for her husband, friends, and relatives. As other people repeatedly fail to meet her expectations, she may develop depression. It is not always easy for the worker to quickly identify a client's cognitive schema. In many circumstances, the worker can gradually come to understand the client's schema through his or her automatic thoughts.

Cognitive Distortions

Cognitive distortions, or automatic thoughts, are the immediate ideas, in the forms of thoughts, images, or internal dialogue and interpretations, that spring to a person's mind (Beck et al., 1979). These thoughts are also called cognitive distortions because they are patterns of cognitive processes that are strongly associated with the ways in which a client customarily misperceives people's intentions and actions (Beck et al., 1979). Certain types of automatic thoughts are commonly found among the depressed clients, and these include:

Selective abstraction. A client selectively chooses and focuses on the negative aspects and ignores the positive aspects of situations and people. For example, a depressed father always complains of his son's unruly behaviors but fails to recognize his son's achievement.

Magnification and minimization. The person magnifies the consequences of a negative event or condition and minimizes his or her own achievements. For example, a student may be extremely upset about getting a C grade in English, but may also ascribe an A grade in mathematics to the leniency of the teacher in marking the examination.

Personalization. This individual assumes responsibility for problems caused by other people. He or she tends to engage in a lot of self-blaming. A depressed mother blames herself for her son's sports injury. She says, "I should have done this or stopped doing that, then my son would not have been hurt." She cannot accept that the injury was an accident that could not be easily prevented.

Absolutist thoughts. The person perceives the rules of life as absolute and engages in a great deal of "mustabatory" thoughts. Life *must* be a certain way. He or she is rigid and cannot easily tolerate ideas that do not fit his or her frame of mind. For example, a depressed man has many mustabatory thoughts about how a father should be treated by his children and how a wife should act toward her husband. When his wife and children do not behave the way he expects them to, he becomes very unhappy.

Interventions Focused on Cognitive Components

Help the client identify and understand his or her pattern of thinking. In many ways, a worker can help a client identify and understand his or her patterns of automatic thoughts and schema that may be linked to his or her depression. The worker can ask the client to do certain exercises such as Beck's (1995) "Daily Record of Dysfunctional Thoughts" worksheet (p. 126). (For an example, see Figure 4.2.) Using such worksheets, the worker can help the client identify his or her automatic thoughts. For example, during an interview, the worker can ask questions such as, "I notice that you hesitated when you were talking about _____. Can you tell me what you were thinking?" or "You seem to have a lot of rules about what it means to be a man. How do these rules affect your life? If you cannot live up to these rules, what does it say about you as an individual?" These questions help the client think about his or her automatic thoughts and schema, and how these cognitive processes may be related to his or her depression.

Help the client think from a different perspective. When a client manifests negative automatic thoughts and rigid rules, the worker can help him or her explore alternative ways of thinking. The purpose is

Date/Time	Situation	Automatic thought(s)	Immediate emotional reaction(s)	Behavioral response(s)
	What was the actual event, thought, or image that triggered your emotions? (e.g., a friend refused to go to a movie with me)	What thought went through your mind? (e.g., he did not treasure our friendship) On a scale of 1 to 10, with 1 being total disbelief and 10 being total belief, how much did you believe your automatic thought was true?	What emotion did you experience at that time? (e.g., anger) From 1 to 10, how intense was your emotion?	How did you respond to the situation? (e.g., walk away) In your opinion, how adaptive or maladaptive was the response?

FIGURE 4.2. Daily Dysfunctional Thoughts Worksheet (*Source:* Adapted from Beck, 1995.)

to help the client to look at an event from a more balanced point of view. This intervention strategy is particularly helpful for a client with depression, because he or she often engages in selective abstraction, personalization, magnification and minimization, and absolutist thoughts. Such an individual believes unwaveringly that his or her thoughts are the correct and only ways to view life. The main objective of this strategy is to help the client learn to entertain the idea that a situation can be seen in more than one way, and that other people in the same situation may have different views. The worker should not force his or her own view onto the client. Rather, he or she should raise questions and ask the client to look at the situation from a different perspective. Examples of the questions may be: "Besides this reason, what other possible reasons do you think can explain this situation?" and "If you are [a person the client knows well], how will he or she see the situation differently?"

Help the client see his or her positives. A client with severe depression does not see anything positives about himself or herself. In fact, the client has only negative views of the future, the world, and himself or herself. During the interview, the worker has to slowly but gradually help the client to look at his or her positives. This is not an easy task, because the client may not be able to see the positives and may feel that the worker does not understand his or her situation. As suggested, the worker should allow the client enough time to ventilate his or her concerns and wait for the right moments to let the client see his or her strengths and the positive aspects of the situation. The worker can use a number of techniques to help the client to examine his or her positives. The worker may use an activity chart to help the client examine the achievement and pleasure he or she gets out of daily activities (Beck, 1995). Essentially, the worker invites the client to record his or her activities and to indicate his or her levels of achievement and of pleasure on a scale of 0 to 5, with 0 being no pleasure and no achievement and 5 being a great deal of pleasurable and achievement (see Figure 4.3). As mentioned, it is more likely that a depressed person will see these events or themselves negatively. The worker's role is to examine the chart together with the client and help him or her evaluate the situation more objectively. For example, the client may say, in general terms, that he or she does not derive any achievement or pleasure from performing certain activities. The worker can invite the client to evaluate these activities objectively and to see whether these activities do, in fact, give him or her little or some achievement

	Day 1	Day 2	Day 3	Day 4	Day 5	Day 6	Day 7
8:00-9:00 a.m.	Breakfast A = 0, P = 2						
9:00-10:00	Did morning excercise A = 1, P = 3	Had a business deal with a client A = 4, P = 4					
10:00-11:00	Went shopping A = 1, P = 3	Talked to the boss A = 0, P = 0					
11:00-12:00 noon	Went shopping A = 1, P = 3						
12:00-1:00 p.m	Had lunch with a good friend A = 2, P = 4						
1:00-2:00	Had lunch with a good friend A = 2, P = 4						
. . .							

FIGURE 4.3. Activity Chart. A (Achievement), 0 = no achievement, 5 = much achievement; P (pleasure), 0 = no pleasure, 5 = much pleasure (*Source:* Adapted from Beck, 1995.)

and pleasure. Clinical experiences show that the client often does not give himself or herself enough credit and fails to appreciate the positives that are present in the process.

The worker may also try to introduce the self-reward exercise (Appendix II), to encourage the client to engage in activities that are rewarding. The worker first encourages the client to think of something (i.e., goals) he or she wants to do before the next counseling session. When these are identified, the client and the worker ouline the specific details about how, when, and where the goals may be achieved. The worker then needs to discuss the kind of rewards the client is going to give himself or herself if the goals are fulfilled. Initially, the worker should encourage the client to think of only easily achievable goals. When the client regains energy and has more confidence, the worker and the client can decide upon other goals. The guiding principle is to enhance the client's success, not his or her failure. In the interview the worker can also point out the positive changes, albeit subtle, that are found in the client. For example, "I notice that you seem to look a bit happier these days. What have you done to make yourself feel happier?" Last, thought-stopping techniques may also be used if the client is troubled by a certain negative thoughts that continue to produce negative emotions. He or she may be taught to recognize these negative thoughts, find some ways of stopping the thoughts, and replace them with positive ones.

Interpersonal and Family Aspects

Family and Friendship Networks

One aspect that affects a person's depressive state is whether he or she has good supportive social and/or family network (Gotlib & Colby, 1987). A depressed client feels lonely and believes that no one understands his or her concerns. Naturally, it is often best if the worker can marshal the support of a client's supportive social and family networks, because the client will feel more supported by his or her "own people" than by others. Indeed, one of the factors in hospitalizing a client is whether the person has a strong supportive network. It is important for the worker to explore if the client has any friends or family members who can help when he or she is feeling down again. One principle in managing a client with severe depression and suicidal ideation is to make sure that the person has company. That individual should not be left alone.

Another issue relating to the family is whether other family members have adequate understanding of depression. Sometimes family members may not understand a client's depression and consider the client's behaviors of apathy and withdrawal as personality problems. This misunderstanding may lead the client to feel rejected and alienated by family members. Moreover, some family members may misunderstand depression as schizophrenia and respond to the client with fear and detachment. It is necessary for the worker to educate family members about depression and about the skills for relating to and helping a relative with depression. However, whereas some family members can be resources for the person with depression, some are not. The worker needs to differentiate the helpful members from the unhelpful members. Otherwise, the unhelpful members can become stressors to the client.

A third issue regarding family members is related to their pent-up feelings. Clinical experiences have shown that some family members experience fear, anxieties, frustrations, and/or anger while they are living with a person suffering from depression. Particularly they feel overwhelmed by the client's issues such as suicide, hospitalization, and a lack of volition. These family members need to express these feelings. Otherwise, they may be at risk of developing poor mental health themselves.

Interpersonal Aspect

Gotlib & Hammen (2002) maintained that a depressed person has an aversive interpersonal style to which others respond with negativity and rejection. His argument stems from the observance that a depressed person quite often exhibits poor social skills: little eye contact, speaks softly and monotonously, and takes a long time to respond to others. His or her conversation is self-focused, negatively toned, and is self-deprecating. Most people are unwilling to engage in a conversation with him or her. The depressed person may then interpret this response as rejection and withdraw from making contact. A vicious cycle begins and the person becomes more socially isolated and withdrawn. This process is referred as the *deviation-amplifying* process (Gotlib & Colby, 1987).

Interventions Focused on Interpersonal and Family Aspects

Social-skills training. Although the role of social-skills deficits in the etiology of depression is not entirely known, social-skills training has been found to improve the interpersonal skills and depressive moods of a client (Hersen, Bellack, & Himmelhoch, 1982). Social-skills training can take the form of basic communication-skills training such as appropriate eye contact, tone of voice, and response time in a conversation. It can also be adopted to train specific interpersonal skills in a given social situation. For example, it can be used to help a depressed person to acquire interpersonal skills for relating to his or her boss and colleagues in the work setting. Video and audio equipment are often used to facilitate the feedback process for the client.

Educating family members. Contents of the education may include the following topics: general knowledge of depression, impacts of depression on the client, medications and side effects, ways of relating to and managing a person with depression, and community resources available to help the client and family members. Such information can be delivered to family members in a group or an individual format.

Facilitating family support groups. While it is helpful for the worker to let family members express their pent-up feelings during individual counseling sessions, it is equally effective to organize family support groups to give family members a platform to air out their concerns. Since family members have similar experiences, support groups can create a sense of comradery among these family members. Moreover, those who have gone through the experiences can share their wisdom with other family members. Indeed, some members may want to talk to people of their "own group" rather than to professionals whom they may consider as distant and unsympathetic.

Linking clients to social and family support. One of the strategies a worker can use is to mobilize interpersonal systems to help the depressed person, particularly if he or she has expressed some suicidal ideas. Sometimes, a severely depressed client may not be able to provide the worker with the names of supportive network members. In such circumstances the worker may need to identify the client's "contact person" (usually available in the medical record) to begin the process of identifying some supportive network members. With the client's permission, the worker can then contact these supportive network members and involve them in the treatment process. Family members are involved in the care of a depressed person and should have a clear understanding of their roles and responsibilities, and they should be trained and supported in carrying out these roles. The idea behind partnership is not about reducing the responsibilities of the mental health worker but about tapping the resources that are most appropriate for the depressed person.

CASE ILLUSTRATION

Background

Mr. Wang was referred to our halfway house by the psychiatric team of a local hospital. His psychiatrist diagnosed him as having major depression and put him on antidepressants. He was hospitalized for about three months after he had tried to commit suicide by starving himself to death. He had been living alone in a hut in New Territories. The psychiatric team felt that Mr. Wang needed further rehabilitation.

Mr. Wang was a fifty-eight-year-old man, and married with a few children. His wife was fifty-four years old and his children were all adults. His wife and children lived in their family home, which was very close to Mr. Wang's hut. Mr. Wang worked in England for twenty-five years and had recently returned to Hong Kong. He had lost all his savings to gambling and was penniless when he came back to Hong Kong. He mentioned that his relationships with his wife and children were distant and that he was somewhat like a stranger to them. He did not have any friends in Hong Kong.

Medical Aspect

Mr. Wang had no family history of depression and had no history of other psychiatric illness. He had no physical problems, except for a minor gastric problem. Preceding hospitalization, he was living with his family members. However, since they could not get along in the family home, he was "forced" to live in the nearby hut. He then started to feel sad, angry, and rejected. He was unable to recall what exactly had happened, only that he began to lose interest in life and withdrew from the world. Even though he realized he was not himself, he did not have the energy to do anything. He said he went into a "deep sleep," and the next thing he knew was that he was in the hospital.

An assessment of his mental state suggested that Mr. Wang was still rather sad and in a low mood. He cried often during interviews and his speech and thought were somewhat slow. He still harbored vague suicide ideation, claiming that he did not find any reason to continue living. In his words, "I have nothing. I deserved to be punished like this. I don't know what I can do." He mentioned that he lost about thirty pounds in the past year and did not have much appetite. However, he slept well enough and was able to engage in conversation. In general, Mr. Wang was still depressed, but was recovering from it.

He was given 150 mg of dothiepin daily. He said he felt better with this medication. Although he experienced side effects of dry mouth and constipation, he did not find these to be serious. He realized he had depression, but did not understand how and why he had it. This provided me with an opportunity to invite him for individual counseling. I gave him information on the biological aspect of depression (verbally and in the form of a booklet for depressed clients) and on the effects and side effects of medication, and I explored with him the impact of psychosocial factors on his depression.

Emotional Aspect

In the initial interviews, Mr. Wang was much overcome by his depression. His blank facial expression, lack of interest in daily life, very soft and slow speech, and crying gave me the impression that he was a very unhappy man. It took only a short while before Mr. Wang began to pour out his life story. He told me of his struggles in England: his busy but lonely life working in Chinatown, the money he sent to his children in Hong Kong, the friends who twice cheated him out of his money, his lost savings, and the gambling problem he acquired a few years before he returned to Hong Kong. He had nothing much left and felt that he was getting old, so he decided to be reunited to his family in Hong Kong. It did not take him long to feel disappointment and unhappiness after his wife and children did not seem to welcome him home. Indeed, he had many unfulfilled expectations relating to the reunion and to a quiet and happy life after retirement. Consequently, he became frustrated, angry, and disillusioned about the people in his life. As a worker, I was prepared to give Mr. Wang as much time as he needed to express his emotions. I was his listener who did not pass judgment onto his behaviors and his life story, nor did I give him any advice as to what he should and should not do. To me, Mr. Wang was yearning to be emotionally connected to someone who was willing to listen to him.

Cognitive Aspect

Mr. Wang obviously had very negative views of himself, of the people around him, and of the future when he was severely depressed. In the interviews, I began to take notice of his negative automatic thoughts. It seemed that he had many absolutist thoughts and personalization. In his words, "I have never been a good father. As a father, I should have spent as much time as I could with them. I should have shown more concern and love for them. I had no excuse," and "I felt I had not been a good husband either. I had left my wife in Hong Kong and spent much time overseas. Why should she love me?" and "I should have known the two fellows better and not be cheated by them; I lost about ten thousand pounds because of the fraud. How stupid was I?" I invited Mr. Wang to explore how these absolutist thoughts and personalization affected his depressed mood. Later, I helped him examine the validity of these thoughts. For example, I asked, "Was it your fault that you had to leave Hong Kong and work in England?" He was able to think and respond that "It was very common for younger man in those days in New Territories to go to England. Money was good there." Essentially, what I tried to do was to raise questions that encouraged Mr. Wang to think through the issues himself. I did not offer him alternative answers.

The predominant schema of Mr. Wang was one of low self-worth. He did not feel he was worthy of any achievements and that he was responsible for creating his worthlessness. Indeed, he tended to claim responsibility for everything that had gone wrong in his life. I helped him examine the evidence for and against his claims, and I helped him explore activities that he could do to make himself feel better. Since he was a chef, it was logical to invite him to help out in the kitchen. Indeed, in the interviews, this appeared to be the only thing that gave Mr. Wang a sense of pride. This turned out to be a good move for Mr. Wang. He felt he was needed in the kitchen and that he was able to do the job well, and he began to feel better about himself and gained some confidence and self-worth.

Interpersonal and Family Aspect

Interpersonal and family relationships were important to Mr. Wang. Unfortunately, in spite of multiple attempts to engage Mr. Wang's family, they were unwilling to participate in the treatment process. In fact, they did not show up for any of the scheduled appointments. Mr. Wang and I discussed this, and he accepted that it was difficult at that time to do anything to improve the family relationship.

In the interpersonal aspect, however, progress could be seen. Mr. Wang began to establish relationships with a few residents in the house, and two residents became important supportive network members for Mr. Wang. They were able to help one another with certain difficulties and needs. Eventually, they decided to apply for public housing together as a group. Since Mr. Wang could be very blunt toward others and made quick assumptions about others' intents, we spent a few sessions discussing how he might improve upon these interpersonal and social skills.

This chapter has highlighted an assessment and intervention framework for working with people suffering from major depression. It is suggested that besides medication, psychosocial interventions are essential in helping a depressed person uplift his or her mood state, understand his or her negative thinking patterns and develop positive and alternative thinking, establish supportive family and friendship networks, and learn social skills. It is important to bear in mind the concept of the cycle of depressed moods (Figure 4.1) and to assess the severity of a client's mood state before venturing into treating the cognitive and behavioral issues related to his or her depression.

Chapter 5

Anxiety Disorders

INTRODUCTION

Anxiety disorders refer to a cluster of anxiety problems, including panic disorder (panicky sensations that appear suddenly, and often without an obvious trigger), generalized anxiety disorder (GAD) (feeling anxious all the time, without a specific source, but can generally be traced back to at least two life events that occur during the six months that the person has the anxious feelings), social or specific phobias (fear of certain objects and social situations), obsessive-compulsive disorder (OCD) (anxiety over uncontrollable thoughts and compulsions), and post-traumatic stress disorder (PTSD) (anxiety over a traumatic experience). The dominant feelings that cut across these disorders are anxiety and fear.

About 14.6 percent of the U.S. population has or has had anxiety problems in their lifetime, and it is the second major mental illness in the United States (Peurifoy, 1995). In Hong Kong, the *Rehabilitation Programme Plan Review* estimates that about 77,400 people suffer from anxiety problems and about 1.5 percent need rehabilitation services (Health and Welfare Bureau, 1999). Another study suggests that anxiety disorders rank first as a major mental illness in Hong Kong (Chen et al., 1993). Similar to depression, many people with anxiety problems receive private medical and psychosocial treatment provided by medical doctors, psychologists, and social workers. Very few are being treated by the mental health care system in Hong Kong.

NATURE OF ANXIETY

Anxiety is a tense emotional state and is often marked by bodily symptoms such as tension, tremor, sweating, and palpitations. It is a reaction to physical or psychological threat (Beck, Emery, & Greenberg, 1985). A person's anxiety state becomes a disorder when the perceived threat (these threats may be anticipatory and may not have actually happened) and/or the associated behavioral responses are excessive and unreasonable (e.g., phobia, OCD), when symptoms are unwanted and unshakable and create psychological distress (e.g., panic attack, GAD), and when the social and/or occupational functioning of the individual is affected. The effect of the disorder on the person's social and/or occupational functioning is localized and confined to specific aspects of his or her life (e.g., a person afraid of heights becomes flooded with anxieties only when he or she is about to enter a high rise).

It is not uncommon for people with anxiety problems to have a secondary or an associated mental illness such as depression. These individuals usually experience very uncomfortable physical symptoms associated with anxiety, and many perceive these anxieties as unpredictable, uncontrollable, and unpleasant. Consequently, they may experience a diminished sense of self-esteem and become depressed. In fact, anxiety problems are often considered as ego-dystonic—despite rationally recognizing their anxieties as excessive and unreasonable, the individuals cannot control these feelings.

ASSESSING A PERSON
WITH ANXIETY PROBLEMS

Figure 5.1 shows the dysfunctional cycle of anxiety disorders. This figure serves as a framework for understanding the anxiety problems faced by a client. Essentially, this cycle suggests that when an individual perceives a stimulus as a threat, he or she will experience physiological sensations such as palpitations, shortness of breath, and sweaty palms. These responses are the body's natural reactions to any perceived threat. These physiological responses then trigger cognitive, behavioral, and emotional responses in an individual. If and when these other responses are maladaptive, the person will become more anxious and fearful when facing the stimulus. A vicious cycle thus ensues. For instance, one of my clients had social phobia and was afraid of going to social gatherings. When she was invited to any social gatherings she would automatically experience physiological sensations of hot flashes, nervousness, and abdominal pain. These

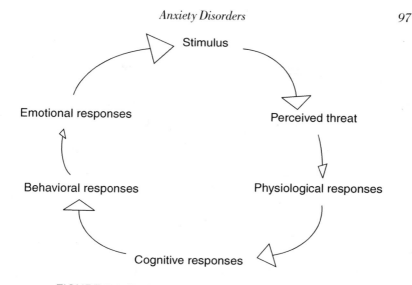

FIGURE 5.1. Dysfunctional Cycle of Anxiety Disorders

uncomfortable feelings triggered her maladaptive cognitive responses such as "I cannot go because I might act stupid in front of my friends." Her maladaptive behavioral response was to avoid going to social gatherings. Unfortunately, the more she declined to go to social gatherings, the worse her condition became. Consequently, she felt very unhappy because she could not cope with her unwanted anxieties. She was very frustrated because she had to make up many excuses to avoid attending social gatherings, and because she felt others considered her as rather odd.

In assessment and intervention it is important for the worker to understand how different parts of this dysfunctional cycle influence a person's anxiety problems. At least four areas should be assessed: (1) medical/physiological, (2) cognitive, (3) behavioral, and (4) emotional aspects.

Medical/Physiological Aspects

Genetic Predisposition

It is useful to find out if any family history of anxiety disorders exists. Although little evidence supports the genetic basis for anxiety problems, studies on twins and families suggest that genes play a role in the origin of anxiety disorders (Kendall & Hammen, 1995). But heredity alone cannot explain the causes of anxiety disorders. Indeed, it can be argued that genetic factors predispose certain people to develop anxiety disorders, and psychosocial and environmental factors contribute to the development of full-blown anxiety disorders (Peurifoy, 1995). In clinical practice it may be useful to provide clients with this information because some of them have misunderstood anxiety disorders as character fraud and blame themselves for causing the anxiety problems. On the other hand, the worker must be very cautious about giving this information to other family members because these family members may become fearful of developing anxiety disorders themselves.

Medical History Related to Anxiety Disorders

It is necessary to first obtain a history of the type of medical treatment the client has received. This includes the types of medications taken, how long the client has been taking the medications, and the dosage of the medications. Although many clients with anxiety disorders do not require hospitalization, it is customary to ask whether he or she has been hospitalized before. This may help the worker discern how well the person has been able to cope with his or her anxiety problem. Since a client may develop withdrawal symptoms as a result of a prolonged intake of antianxiety medications, it is particularly important to review the kinds of medications he or she has been taking, and to find out whether the client has adequate understanding of the effects and side effects of the medications. In addition, some clients who have become dependent on certain antianxiety medications may engage in doctor-shopping behaviors or go to different drugstores to buy the medications. These medications are not supposed to be taken for an extended period of time, as they may lead to harmful and prolonged drug dependence. The worker should explore whether his or her clients have these doctor-shopping and drug-shopping behaviors.

It is difficult but useful and important to clearly unearth the underlying stressors that cause anxiety disorders. For example, a client with PTSD would have experienced a traumatic event, and, as a result, developed various anxiety symptoms. It is important for the worker to thoroughly examine the types of stressors that may be closely linked to clients with PTSD and other anxiety disorders.

Other Medical or Psychiatric Causes of Anxiety Symptoms

People suffering from medical conditions such as cardiovascular problems, asthma, hyperthyroidism, and problems with inner ears, and from psychiatric conditions such as psychotic state and mania may also experience anxiety symptoms (American Psychiatric Association, 2000). It is essential for the mental health worker to ask the client whether he or she has any of these conditions or whether he or she has consulted medical doctors regarding these conditions. The worker should encourage the client to consult a medical doctor if he or she thinks that the client may be suffering from any of these conditions, and may not have a genuine anxiety problem. For example, a female client of mine who was initially diagnosed to be suffering from panic disorder was later found to have angina. Not only was she spared the medications, and thus the side effects of medications, she was also relieved from bearing a label of being mentally ill. As a business executive, she was quite worried about how her colleagues might see her should they know that she might be suffering from a mental disorder. Indeed, a misdiagnosis may aggravate the medical and psychiatric condition, creating unnecessary suffering for the individual concerned.

Secondary Depression

As previously mentioned, it is quite common for people with an anxiety disorder to be suffering from depression as well. Although the primary diagnosis is still anxiety disorder, depression as a secondary diagnosis should also be medically treated. The mental health worker should periodically examine whether a client with anxiety disorder is becoming depressed. Although the worker needs to inform the psychiatrist of the change in the client's mental state, he or she should carefully tap into the client's mood state in order to detect any suicidal ideations.

Severity of Anxiety Disorders:
Mental State Examination

The severity of anxiety disorders is determined by (1) duration of symptoms/illness, (2) impacts of the illness on the social and occupational functioning, and (3) insight into illness and compliance with medications.

Number of symptoms and duration of illness. The number of symptoms and duration of symptom manifestations are different for different anxiety disorders (American Psychiatric Association, 2000). For example, a person who is diagnosed as suffering from panic disorder experiences recurrent and intense fear and discomfort. This is accompanied by at least four or more other symptoms (listed in the DSM-IV-TR) over a very short period of ten minutes. He or she will also experience panic attacks several times a week or several times a day (American Psychiatric Association, 2000). Generalized anxiety disorder (GAD) is another example. The essential characteristics of GAD are excessive anxiety and worry (apprehensive expectation), occurring for a period of at least six months and associated with a number of stressful daily concerns such as finances and health of family members (American Psychiatric Association, 2000). It is important for the mental health worker to be familiar with the different criteria and be able to ask relevant questions that help draw some initial understanding of the type of anxiety disorder suffered by the client.

Impacts on social and occupational functioning. If the person manifests symptoms of an anxiety disorder that do not significantly affect his or her functioning (e.g., ability to perform job), he or she may not be considered as having a severe anxiety disorder. Those who are clinically anxious are unable to perform certain social and occupational roles that he or she can normally do.

Case Example. Joe developed intense fear and worries of leaving his apartment and locked himself inside for the past two months. Whenever he thought of leaving his house he became very worried, experiencing palpitations, rapid breathing, ideas of flight, and fears of fainting and dying. As a consequence, his relatives had to bring him food and did all the household chores for him. Not surprising, he had to request sick leave and his employment was disrupted for more than a month.

Insight into illness/compliance to medications. People with anxiety disorders are usually aware of their illnesses. As a matter of fact, many are quite concerned about the absurdity of their symptoms, and are frustrated by their lack of ability to control their anxieties. To a greater extent, due to these frustrations, some may develop depression as a secondary illness. It is sometimes useful to guide a client to accept the absurdity of his or her anxiety problem (e.g., a specific phobia). When they can be more accepting of the illness, they will be less anxious.

Although hospitalization is rarely required for a person with an anxiety disorder, it is sometimes useful to ask the client whether he or she has ever received hospitalization, particularly if the client has secondary depression. A worker should also determine whether psychotropic medications or counseling is a better option for the client. The worker should examine each option carefully. Medications are often prescribed to help the client to feel less anxious, but medications alone cannot address the underlying issues causing the anxiety. In many circumstances, both medications and counseling are needed. Medications can reduce clients' anxieties, and counseling can help them work through troubling issues and learn skills to manage their anxiety symptoms.

Medical Treatments

Drug treatment. Benzodiazepines such as Xanax, clonazepam, and valium relieve symptoms quickly and have few side effects, although drowsiness can be a problem (Sundel & Sundel, 1998). Benzodiazepines include clonazepam, which is used for social phobia and GAD; alprazolam, which is helpful for panic disorder and GAD; and lorazepam, which is also useful for panic disorder. Buspirone is a newer antianxiety medication that is used to treat GAD. Unlike the benzodiazepines, buspirone must be taken consistently for at least two weeks to achieve the antianxiety effect. In addition to the side effects such as drowsiness and dizziness, some people can develop a tolerance to benzodiazepines (i.e., they would have to continue increasing the dosage to get the same effect). Therefore, benzodiazepines are generally prescribed for short periods of time. One exception is panic disorder, for which they may be used for six months to a year. People who have had problems with drug or alcohol abuse may not be suitable candidates for these medications because they may become dependent on them.

Some people experience withdrawal symptoms when they stop taking benzodiazepines. Gradually reducing the dosage can decrease the likelihood of such symptoms occurring. In certain instances, the symptoms of anxiety can rebound after these medications are stopped. Potential problems with benzodiazepines have led some physicians to shy away from using them, or to use them in inadequate doses, even when they are of potential benefit to the client.

A number of medications that were originally used for treatment of depression have been found to be effective for anxiety disorders. SSRIs (selective serotonin reuptake inhibitors) such as fluoxetine and sertraline are commonly prescribed for people who have panic disorder in combination with OCD, social phobia, or depression (U.S. Public Health Service, 2004). Venlafaxine, a drug very similar to an SSRI, is useful for treating GAD. These medications are started at a low dose and are gradually increased until they reach a therapeutic level.

Similarly, antidepressant medications called tricyclics are useful in treating people with co-occurring anxiety disorders and depression. Clomipramine, the only antidepressant in its class prescribed for OCD, and imipramine, prescribed for panic disorder and GAD, are examples of tricyclics (U.S. Public Health Service, 2004). As for MAOIs (monoamine oxidase inhibitors), the most commonly prescribed MAOI is phenelzine, which is helpful for people with panic disorder and social phobia. People who take MAOIs are put on a restrictive diet because these medications can interact with some foods and beverages, including cheese and red wine (U.S. Public Health Service, 2004). Interactions between MAOIs and other substances can cause dangerous elevations in blood pressure or other potentially life-threatening reactions. The worker needs to remind the client that antidepressants take several weeks before they take effect. It is important for the client not to get discouraged and stop taking these medications at too early a stage of the medical intervention.

Educating the client. This point is based on the assumption that a biological basis exists for the occurrence of anxiety symptoms and that some people can become stressed and anxious more easily than others. Simply put, physiological responses to threat are a natural process as an attempt to guard against personal danger. Physiological arousal actually prepares the organism to engage in the fight or flight response. However, the sympathetic nervous system (responsible for physiological arousal) is more easily aroused in some individuals and cannot be adequately balanced by the activation of the parasympathetic nervous system (responsible for restoring the arousal to a balanced state). A worker who adheres to a biopsychosocial perspective may suggest that some people can become more easily anxious than others due to biological reasons. This strategy may be particularly useful for clients with panic disorder and GAD because it will help them to feel "normalized" and feel that their anxiety is not caused by character problems or unhappy childhood and life experiences.

For example, a sixty-year-old woman who had panic disorder often associated her anxieties with the poor relationships she had with her mother during childhood. Although this connection may or may not be true, it stopped her from devoting energy to learn ways of managing her symptoms. Indeed, she continued to blame her anxieties and present inadequacies on her childhood experiences. An understanding of the biological basis of anxiety helped this woman look at her anxiety problem differently, and it lessened her unhappiness and sense of powerlessness in changing her situation. It is also useful for the worker to provide some reading materials such as a fact sheet on anxiety disorders to his or her clients, and to encourage clients to read these materials on their own.

The worker also needs to educate his or her clients on the possible link between physiological responses and other response systems. It is often helpful to present the model of dysfunctional cycle of anxiety disorders (Figure 5.1) to clients, and ask them to use their own examples to analyze whether such links exist. When they are able to see the connections among these response systems, the worker can then encourage the clients to derive strategies to manage their physiological symptoms.

Strategies for symptom management. It is important to remind the client that the earlier anxiety symptoms are recognized and managed, the easier it is to stop the dysfunctional cycle and gain a sense of control.

1. The first step is to help the client to recognize his or her pattern of maladaptive physiological symptoms. One way of doing this is to ask the client to think of and focus on an anxiety-provoking situation. The worker then encourages the client to remember the different physiological symptoms he or she is reexperienc-

ing. Another way of doing this is to ask the client to fill out a physiological symptom checklist (Appendix III). It is important to ask the client to mark the most common physiological symptoms he or she experiences in different situations. The main idea with either technique is to help the client identify his or her pattern of physiological responses. Clinical experiences show that each client has his or her unique pattern of physiological responses, and it is helpful for him or her to recognize and find ways of managing them.

2. The second step in the process is to ask the client to rate the degree of discomfort associated with the presence of these symptoms (0 = no discomfort, 10 = extreme discomfort).

3. The third step is to introduce breathing exercises or relaxation exercises (imagery or muscle relaxation) to the client. The worker should let the client practice as many times as needed until he or she has mastered the exercises. It is not necessary for the client to learn the full set of imagery or relaxation exercises. Rather, the client needs to learn only a few that can be used whenever he or she faces anxiety-provoking situations.

4. When the client has learned all the steps, the worker can ask the client to go through the entire process by focusing on an anxiety-provoking situation, recognizing his or her pattern of physiological symptoms, rating the degree of discomfort, practicing a partial breathing or relaxation exercise, and rating the degree of discomfort after the exercise is used. The worker should remind the client that it takes time to master the skills, and that practice is important.

Physiological Symptoms

Physiological symptoms are an important area of assessment because they are the very first stage of the dysfunctional cycle of anxiety disorders (see Figure 5.1). According to Figure 5.1, physiological sensations associated with an anxiety disorder serve as automatic alarm signals that trigger other dysfunctional response systems. It is not uncommon to find that some clients can recount in vivid detail their physiological sensations when they are feeling anxious. These symptoms are often experienced as unpleasant sensations that continuously bombard the individuals: shortness of breath, choking, heartburn, nausea, etc. These sensations are unwanted and unshakable. Individuals experiencing these physiological sensations simply cannot "switch them off" when they are turned on. Such lack of control is distressing and frustrating to the client.

With time, these individuals appear to become hypervigilant about the physiological sensations. As soon as they experience any physiological changes they begin to assume the worst. For example, one of my clients mentioned that whenever she enters a crowded and stuffy environment, such as on a bus, she immediately feels choking sensations and hot flashes. She starts to feel panicky, and predicts that she is going to suffocate and die. Consequently, her dysfunctional cycle of anxiety begins to roll automatically. If others similar to my client can develop strategies to relieve and gain a sense of control over these physiological symptoms, the dysfunctional cycle may come to a stop. Thus, it is necessary for the worker to help the client recognize his or her idiosyncratic physiological alarm signals and to develop cognitive and behavioral strategies to relieve these physiological symptoms. In Chapter 4, in the discussion on depression, emotions were mentioned as the initial point of intervention. For anxiety disorders, the initial point of intervention centers on the management of physiological symptoms. The ability to manage the physiological symptoms may reduce a client's physical and psychological discomfort, and it can also help the client develop a sense of control over the symptoms, thus inducing a sense of confidence.

Cognitive Aspects

According to Beck et al. (1985), three main components in the cognitive process are related to the clients' anxiety problems: negative automatic thoughts, intermediate beliefs, and negative core beliefs (intermediate beliefs and core beliefs are often grouped under the umbrella term *schema,* as for depression as discussed in Chapter 4).

Automatic Thoughts

The contents of these immediate thoughts for someone suffering from an anxiety disorder are negative, anticipatory, and seemingly uncontrollable, and the distortions are linked to five cognitive processes: catastrophic thoughts, absolutist thoughts, fortune-telling, magnification and minimization, and negative self-talk.

Catastrophic thoughts. This is a common habit among people with anxiety problems. They anticipate that something disastrous is going to happen and they will consequently be physically endangered or socially embarrassed. For example, one of my clients believed that if she took a certain turn at a particular street, she would get into a fatal accident (however, she had no previous experience of this). Another client suggested that she would suffocate or die of a heart attack if she entered a crowded place. Such catastrophic thoughts create intense fear. Although some clients understand that the thoughts are groundless, they cannot get rid of the fear.

Absolutist thoughts. Individuals with anxiety disorders are rather rigid in thinking and see life in absolute terms. They are preoccupied with certain thoughts and cannot entertain other possibilities. People with OCD are extreme examples of such thought patterns, though the habit is not exclusive to OCD sufferers. People with various types of anxiety disorders have very rigid thinking as well.

Case example. Miss Hung saw everything as black and white and would adhere to her views unswervingly. What she believed was true and right and all other views were wrong. She thought that fish reared in ponds were toxic, and she would ask restaurant staff in detail about the origins of the fish available on the menu. Also she felt that her hands might catch the germs in the air and be fatal to her health, so she wore gloves every day, rain or shine.

Fortune-telling. This is a common thought pattern found among people with anxiety disorders. They tend to predict negative outcomes and start to worry about issues long before they happen, if they happen at all. Indeed, many are able to describe their predictions in vivid detail, and they assume these outcomes to be the only possible outcomes. As a result they become very anxious.

Case example. Mr. Liu had to make an oral presentation at work in front of his colleagues and boss. He mentioned in detail the silly mistakes he was sure he would make during the presentation—he would stutter, forget to bring the written scripts, the computer would break down, people would not listen and get bored, etc. He became so preoccupied with these thoughts that he did not have the energy to prepare for the presentation.

Magnification and minimization. Unlike some clients who anticipate that something disastrous is going to happen, clients with the habit of magnification and minimization magnify the consequences of a current situation and minimize their ability to handle the situation. Thus, they become very anxious. For example, a student taking an examination perceived the exam as the determining factor of his future career when in reality it was just a midyear exam (maximization). He also felt that he could not pass the exam (minimization). This created a great deal of anxiety for him.

Negative self-talk. Some clients engage in negative self-dialogue that is discouraging and destructive. Two possible themes relate to this negative self-talk: inadequate control and coping (e.g., "I can't do it. I cannot stop it from happening"), and self-blaming (e.g., "I should have spent more time doing it. I should have been able to deal with it"). This dialogue pops up when the clients face anxiety-provoking situations, further aggravating the anxieties experienced by these individuals.

Intermediate Beliefs

Whereas automatic thoughts are images and words that occur when an individual is faced with anxiety-provoking situations, intermediate beliefs are often manifested as dysfunctional rules, which are rigid guidelines and dogmas that strongly influence the person's perception and judgment about certain issues and practices. These dysfunctional rules influence automatic thoughts. For example, a man may strongly believe that it is his responsibility to earn money to feed his family, and that a woman should be a housewife and take care of the children. He may experience tremendous stress if, for example, he hears rumors that his company is going to lay off workers and that he may become jobless. An individual with an anxiety disorder has many rigid rules. Although it is difficult to recall where and how the individual acquires such rules, it may be traced to a person's childhood socialization, particularly from his or her family. The tendency is that the more rigid a person's rules, the more negative his or her negative emotions will be because the reality does not concur with one's rules and expectations. Moreover, some of these rules are principles that guide a person's perceptions and actions and may lead to interpersonal conflicts with others. Clients may express the following rules:

- When offering certain opinions, they may utter "should/must" statements, particularly regarding issues related to family roles and social roles. For example, a man may say "A father should be respected by his son, and the son cannot talk back to the father."
- These rules then manifest into "if-then" statements. For example, "If I don't work hard, then I'll flunk the course," "If I do poorly on the presentation then my boss will not trust me," "If I raise differences, I won't be loved," and "If I can't control my fear, everyone will notice it and laugh at me." These are conditional statements that are often interpreted by clients as imperative, and as rules by which they consciously and unconsciously require themselves to live.

Core Beliefs

Core beliefs refer to one's evaluation of and underlying beliefs about oneself (Beck et al., 1985). People with anxiety disorders tend to have negative core beliefs related to one or more of the following three themes: acceptance (e.g., "I don't deserve love"), competence (e.g., "I am inadequate"), and control (e.g., "Nothing is in my control"). Core beliefs affect one's confidence and perpetuate the dysfunctional cycle of anxiety disorders. For example, a client may see himself or herself as inadequate, imperfect, or weak. This negative self-evaluation affects the client's confidence and makes him or her feel powerless and insecure when faced with an anxiety-provoking situation. Consequently, the person may become more anxious. Core beliefs are at the very center of a client's cognitive distortion process, and may not be easily recognized by the worker. Normally, core beliefs are manifested through a person's dysfunctional rules and automatic thoughts. For example, if a person holds the core belief that "I'm not good enough," the intermediate belief may be, "Even if I work hard, I still cannot compete with others." The automatic thoughts that may be related to this core belief are "I can't do it" (absolutist thought), and "why should I even bother to try? I'll make a fool of myself" (self-talk or fortune-telling). In the counseling process the worker and client should examine these intermediate beliefs and automatic thoughts closely so that they can identify the client's core belief. Sometimes, it may take a while before they can clearly identify the underlying core belief.

Interventions Focusing on Cognitive Aspects

Help the client identify automatic thoughts and how they are linked to anxieties. The worker can make use of a worksheet similar to Beck's (1995) "Daily Record of Dysfunctional Thoughts" worksheet (p. 126) (see Figure 4.2 in Chapter 4) to help the client record several anxiety-provoking situations, and then review the various physiological, cognitive, emotional, and behavioral responses associated with the client's anxiety-provoking situations. The worker can guide the client in finding his or her unique automatic thoughts and behavioral patterns as well as help the client understand the link between these responses. Indeed, it is important for the client to clearly accept that cognition affects his or her behavioral and emotional responses.

Help the client control automatic thoughts. One of the techniques that may be useful for controlling automatic thoughts is called *thought stopping.* The following list describes the six steps for using this technique:

Step 1: Identify situations that frequently produce anxiety for the client (e.g., facing bosses and colleagues at work).

Step 2: Identify the negative automatic thoughts related to the anxiety-provoking situations (e.g., "I am going to be scolded by my boss again" or "I am going to make a fool of myself in front of my colleagues").

Step 3: Ask the client to imagine the situation and to say *stop* when the specific anxiety-provoking situation emerges (e.g., Imagine getting ready for work, then say *stop* when the thought "I am going to be scolded by my boss again" occurs).

Step 4: Identify positive coping statements to counteract the negative automatic thoughts (e.g., "What is the worst that can happen to me? All bosses are like that").

Step 5: Ask the client to rate, from 1 to 10, how he or she feels after using a positive coping statement.

Step 6: Repeat the first five steps until the client is able to re-place the negative automatic thoughts with a positive coping statement as naturally as possible. Sometimes it is helpful to teach the client a breathing technique to help him or her first calm down before trying the positive coping statement. More-over, some clients find it useful to write positive coping state-ments on cue cards. Whenever they face the identified anxiety-provoking situations they can take the card out as a visual reminder to practice the positive coping statements.

Examine the validity of dysfunctional rules. A worker can help the client examine the validity of his or her dysfunctional rules in a num-ber of ways, two methods being cognitive restructuring and behav-ioral experimentation.

Cognitive restructuring: Invite a client to examine evidence for or against his or her claims. Moreover, a client can also be helped to evaluate the consequence of a certain claim. For ex-ample, a client who believes that a man who does not earn an income is not a real man can be asked to list names of men who are breadwinners, but who the client thinks are not real men. In addition to drawing evidence for or against one's view, it is useful to ask if the client knows someone who may have a different view. The worker can follow this by asking the client how this person might see the situation differently. Last, for a client who frequently engages in catastrophic thoughts, it is useful to ask him or her to describe the worst scenario that can possibly happen, and on a scale of 1 to 10 (1 = being totally impossible and 10 = being totally possible), rank to what extent he or she believes it will occur.

Behavioral experimentation: Invite the client to examine the va-lidity of his or her beliefs by collecting evidence in daily life to support or dispute his or her dysfunctional beliefs. Behav-ioral experimentation is different from cognitive restructur-ing in that behavioral experimentation requires the client to engage in an exercise to collect evidence for or against his or her beliefs, whereas cognitive restructuring is a mental activ-

ity. For example, a man who believes that his son should behave in a certain way or else become an inadequate man can
ask other fathers whether his claim is true. However, the
worker needs to discuss, in detail, how, where, and when the
client will conduct the experiment. Moreover, the client needs
to identify what evidence will be considered as supporting or
refuting the claim. This procedure should be exercised with
care and tact in order to maximize the learning opportunity.

Help the client modify core beliefs. Core beliefs are most resistant
to change. Since it has taken a long time and many experiences for a
client to develop core beliefs, a great deal of evidence and experience
is required for the client to change these core beliefs. The central intervention focus is to provide as much evidence as possible for why
the client should and can change his or her self-perception. The following list offers a number of ways that can facilitate this changing
process:

- By using the dysfunctional thoughts worksheet (see Figure 4.2
  in Chapter 4), the worker can help the client identify his or her
  core beliefs and help him or her connect these core beliefs to automatic thoughts and dysfunctional rules. The worker can help
  the client to identify the core beliefs that are manifested in the
  client's automatic thoughts and dysfunctional rules. The client
  needs to understand and agree upon the connection. This is essentially achieved by helping the client fill out a case conceptualization map (Beck, 1995). (For an example, see Figure 5.2.)
- Many clients may feel that their core beliefs are so deeply rooted
  that it would be impossible to modify them. The worker can help
  the client consider the negative consequences of holding onto
  such beliefs and encourage him or her to realize that it is simply
  a matter of personal choice whether to hold onto or change the
  beliefs. I often ask this question: "If you realize how your core
  beliefs are negatively affecting your life, why is it worth holding
  onto them?"
- An activity chart that contains a breakdown of the day into hours
  and extends over a week is another tool that can be used to help
  modify core beliefs (Beck, 1995) (see Figure 4.3 in Chapter 4).
  The client is encouraged to fill out the worksheet daily and to in-

dicate the major activities that have occurred. The activities should be rated in terms of pleasure (1 = not pleasurable, 5 = extremely pleasurable) and accomplishment (1 = no accomplishment, 5 = complete accomplishment). The worker can then go through the worksheet and encourage the client to increase the activities that gave pleasure and accomplishment. With time this practice can help the client create a balanced and positive lifestyle.

- Self-reward exercises help the client develop and carry out the action plans (see Appendix II). The worker needs to discuss the weekly short-term goals in detail with the client. The goals should be specific and achievable, and the criteria for success should also be clearly spelled out. The worker should also help the client identify "rewards" to give himself or herself when a stated goal has been achieved.

Behavioral Aspects

Assessment

Some clients with anxiety disorders engage in self-defeating behaviors (maladaptive coping behaviors) that further perpetuate the anxieties they are experiencing. Paradoxically, these self-defeating behaviors are used by clients as methods to help reduce their levels of anxiety or discomfort. When these behaviors are repeatedly reinforced they become automatic behavioral responses that are difficult to unlearn. For example, a man with social phobia and panic attack may turn to alcohol to help him relax, feeling that as soon as he has a drink he will feel less anxious. Thus, whenever he is faced with an anxiety-provoking situation he resorts to drinking. The drinking will consequently lead to more problems that will only increase his anxieties, unless the worker helps him properly develop adaptive strategies and skills to deal with the anxiety-provoking situations and his anxiety symptoms.

Interventions

The main focuses of interventions are (1) to help the client replace maladaptive behaviors with adaptive ones and (2) to desensitize the person to the anxiety-provoking situations.

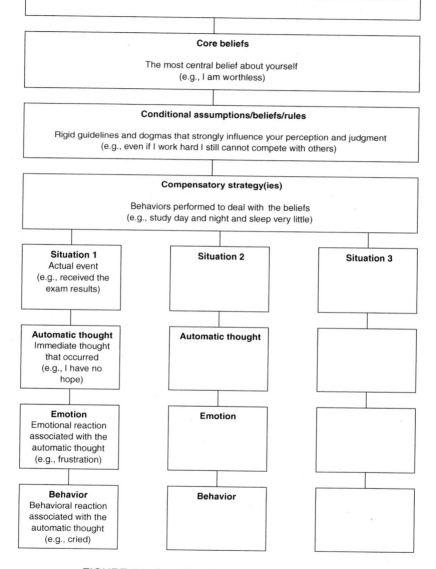

FIGURE 5.2. Cognitive Conceptualization Diagram

Replace self-defeating behaviors. Coping-skills training is one way of helping the client learn new coping behaviors. To begin with, the worker helps the client understand the links between the anxiety-provoking situations, self-defeating behaviors, and his or her anxiety. When the client is able to understand these links, the worker and the client identify other alternative and adaptive coping skills that the client can use when he or she faces such situations. The client should rate the degree of probable usefulness of each of these alternative coping behaviors on a scale of 1 to 10 (1 = not useful, 10 = most useful). The worker needs to help the client find ways in which he or she may carry out adaptive coping behaviors along with the possible obstacles that he or she will encounter in the process.

Case example. Mr. Lam would experience panic sensations when he was alone at home, particularly in the afternoon. Immediately, he would resort to drinking alcohol to soothe his anxieties. Mr. Lam and his therapist discussed how his anxieties and self-defeating behaviors were reinforced—not soothed—by his drinking, and came up with a few alternative coping behaviors. Mr. Lam decided to go for a walk in the nearby park whenever he started experiencing a panic attack. He would walk for at least half an hour, then rate his level of anxiety to distinguish whether the walking helped.

Desensitize the client. If the client's anxiety is related to a specific object or situation, graded exposure is a technique that can help the client to desensitize himself or herself to the situation or object. The worker and the client should explore the degrees of anxiety associated with the various conditions relating to an object or a situation. For example, a client is asked to rate his different levels of anxiety associated with the image of his boss, of his boss approaching him, and of talking with his boss face to face. When this is completed, the worker should help the client learn to practice relaxation with the image of his boss in mind. Once he is able to feel relaxed about this image, he moves on to the next image of his boss approaching him. This process continues until the client is able to talk to his boss directly without feeling anxious.

Emotional Aspects

The emotional aspects of the dysfunctional cycle of anxiety disorder that are targeted during assessment and intervention are: (1) fear of fear, and (2) emotions as outcomes of anxiety problems.

Assessment

Fear of fear. The experience of anxiety is often so highly distressing to the person that it generates a second level of fear: the person becomes afraid of becoming afraid. He or she dreads experiencing the anxiety symptoms and becomes anxious and hypervigilant of the symptoms. This constant worry over avoiding anxiety symptoms is what actually causes anxiety symptoms, such as choking sensations, palpitations, and revulsions. Moreover, the fear of being seen by others as being anxious makes the person even more anxious. For example, a client of mine had developed the fear that he spit when he talked. He became very sensitive to this sensation and was hypervigilant of any indication given by the person to whom he was speaking that he had spit. He believed that any time someone touched their face or moved slightly during conversation was because he had spit on them. He began holding his hand in front of his mouth when he talked, causing him to seem even more abnormal to those with whom he spoke and thus increasing his anxiety. Because his anxiety caused him to behave strangely, he became anxious of becoming anxious. He became so anxious of his anxieties that he began avoiding conversation altogether. The fear of experiencing anxieties generates a great deal more anxieties for many individuals.

Emotions. Generally speaking, under this framework of dysfunctional cycle, emotions are considered to be outcomes of the disorders. Other factors, such as cognition, are responsible for inducing anxieties and other emotions in the client. As mentioned, the client may experience a gamut of emotions such as depressed moods, shame, guilt, and fear. The worker needs to take notice of these emotions and respond by helping the client fully express them.

Interventions

Help the client to fully express his or her anxieties by creating a warm and accepting therapeutic relationship. The worker is advised to use such skills as active listening, empathy, and unconditional positive regard to facilitate the development of such a relationship.

Help the client to accept his or her anxieties. Many clients with anxiety disorders feel powerless to control their anxieties and become very frustrated and fearful. They cannot accept that anxieties are natural human responses to perceived threats and believe that the presence of anxieties is unacceptable. A helpful strategy to use in the initial stage of intervention is to educate clients about the biological nature of anxiety. Some clients tend to be more relaxed when they realize that it is normal to be anxious.

CASE ILLUSTRATION

Shirley was a thirty-two-year-old married woman. She was living in a self-owned apartment with her husband, her father-in-law, and her mother-in-law. She described her husband as a responsible and loving man but saw her in-laws as somewhat difficult to live with. She would keep herself fully occupied in the evenings so that she would not have to eat dinner with her in-laws. She had been diagnosed as having generalized anxiety disorder. She worked as a clerk in a business firm in Hong Kong and her husband worked in mainland China, returning home on the weekends. She continued to receive medical treatment from her psychiatrist, and came to see me for counseling.

Medical Aspect

Shirley had no family history of anxiety disorder, nor did she suffer from another medical or psychiatric illness. (This was confirmed by the psychiatrist.) She developed anxiety symptoms about two years prior to starting treatment with me. She experienced palpitations, choking sensations, sweaty palms, loss of appetite, hot and cold spells, and derealization. It came to a point that small and simple occurrences could trigger an episode of anxiety, and it would take her a week or more to become calm again. About two months before she came to see me, her anxiety episodes had become much more frequent, and she felt she had been taking too many sick leaves from work. She did not understand why she had such anxiety problems, and felt rather uncomfortable with and fearful of the symptoms.

A number of life-changing events had happened during the time in which her anxiety symptoms began. First, her husband had started working in mainland China. Second, they moved in with her in-laws. Third, her job situation was insecure and rumors were being spread about her employers downsizing the company. These factors no doubt contributed to Shirley's anxiety.

Shirley was put on alprazolam, but described this and other antianxiety medications she took as ineffective. She did not experience any side effects from the medication, and was not aware of the possible withdrawal symptoms. She had adequate insight into her illness and was compliant to the medications. Since she wanted to get pregnant, her goal was to eliminate her need for medication.

Since Shirley could easily fall into her dysfunctional cycle of anxiety problems, the first thing she and I did together was explore her pattern of physiological responses. This was done to help her quickly recognize that she might fall into the cycle again. Choking sensations, palpitations, and sweaty palms were the three physiological symptoms that often accompanied Shirley's anxieties. I taught her to use simple breathing techniques whenever she recognized these symptoms. I also gave Shirley a booklet on anxiety disorders.

Cognitive Aspect

Shirley was a fairly typical individual with the habits of catastrophic thoughts and fortune-telling. Throughout the initial stage of the counseling process, Shirley described many situations she encountered as disastrous and made ungrounded assumptions about future happenings. For example, in one of the interviews Shirley told me that her sister mentioned that she was financially "tight." Shirley became very anxious and could not calm herself down for a week. She thought, "I hope my sister is not in debt. It is not easy to deal with the loan shark, and we will all be in trouble," "I cannot lend her my savings. I need the money myself," "If mother knows that she is in debt, she would be heartbroken. I cannot let Mom become miserable," and "She [her sister] has never learned to control her spending. I have warned her so many times." These thoughts kept repeating themselves and occupied her mind day and night.

During the process, I invited Shirley to record when her dysfunctional thoughts occurred and how they made her feel. We then explored how these thoughts were related to other aspects of the dysfunctional cycle. She quickly realized that her catastrophic thoughts contributed much to her anxieties, and that the situations might not be as disastrous as she thought. However, she still found it difficult to stop these automatic thoughts. My strategy was to help Shirley recognize these catastrophic thoughts as early as she could and to help her "stop" the thoughts before they became uncontrollable. Gradually, she was able to recognize that she engaged in these thoughts and consciously tried to stop herself by naming these thoughts as catastrophic.

Shirley had many dysfunctional rules, both in the forms of "if-then" and "should" statements. For example, she tried to keep herself fully occupied with activities. She spent many nights learning accounting and various computer programs, and she even used her lunchtime to learn conversational English. In her words, "If I do not equip myself, then I will be the first to go" (even though her performance had been quite good, as she later told me), "Even if I tried very hard, others performed better than me," "It is my responsibility as a worker to do the best I can" and "I must finish my works far ahead of time to have time to correct the mistakes I'll make." Although some of these statements could be interpreted as positive, Shirley did not allow these rules much flexibility. As a consequence, she became very tense and uptight. When Shirley discussed these rules with me, it became apparent that she had always evaluated herself as inadequate (core beliefs). She tried very hard to overcome her perceived inadequacies, but tended to look for further inadequacies rather than recognizing her achievements. Consequently, her core beliefs were reinforced.

I invited Shirley to record her daily activities. She realized that she was "on the go" all the time and did not give herself enough time to rest. Moreover, she did not give herself enough credit for her accomplishments and often minimized her achievements. We decided to use self-reward exercises and set periodic short-term goals for Shirley. After a few trials, Shirley was able to set realistic goals for herself and began to acknowledge and to give credit to her achievements. Indeed, Shirley gained more confidence about herself.

Behavioral Aspect

Shirley's major self-defeating behaviors concerned (1) a heavy reliance on medication when she felt anxious and (2) reliance on her mother to provide words of comfort. In fact, when she felt anxious, she would immediately take medication and go home to visit her mother. Although she was able to get a sense of relief by doing this, she had never learned to develop strategies to manage and prevent her anxiety symptoms. Shirley and I discussed alternative adaptive coping behaviors that she might want to use to handle her anxieties. She decided to use a breathing technique to soothe her anxieties, and to write her concerns in a daily log book and to spend a certain time in the evening to think about them. She was asked to rate the severity of the issues and to consider whether she had engaged in any dysfunctional automatic thoughts.

Since Shirley's busy lifestyle was somewhat related to her ongoing anxieties, we discussed how she might maintain a more balanced lifestyle. She decided to cut down on her activities in the evenings and was willing to spend more time at home with her in-laws. She would put aside a certain time in the evening as her "quiet time" to use as she pleased. Her activity chart revealed that she spent a great deal of time in employment-related activities, thus she was encouraged to allocate more time to other pleasurable social activities. She decided to devote a bit more time to talking with her in-laws and to social activities with a group of friends.

Emotional Aspect

Initially, Shirley was very much overwhelmed by her anxieties and felt herself to be powerless in handling these anxieties. Although I could not detect any major depressive symptoms in her, she was quite distressed by her anxieties. Through active listening, empathy, and unconditional positive regard, I tried to create a warm atmosphere in which Shirley could fully express her emotions. It seemed as though Shirley felt very comfortable with me and was willing to fully participate in the counseling process.

This chapter has highlighted an assessment and intervention framework for working with people suffering from anxiety problems. The dysfunctional cycle of anxiety disorders suggests that intervention should first be focused on helping an individual acquire a sense of control over uncomfortable physiological responses, then, when the person's level of anxiety is reduced, the intervention focus may then be shifted to helping him or her deal with the maladaptive cognitive, behavioral, and emotional responses. It is helpful to utilize a case conceptualization diagram to understand the interrelationships between the various responses to better help treat clients suffering from anxiety disorders.

Chapter 6

Schizophrenia

INTRODUCTION

Schizophrenia is a major psychotic disorder. It is characterized by the presence of positive and negative symptoms such as delusions, hallucinations, disorganized speech, grossly disorganized and catatonic behaviors, and poor self-care. A person who is diagnosed as having schizophrenia must have psychotic disturbances that last for at least six months and include at least one month of active-phase symptoms (delusions, hallucinations, negative symptoms, etc.) (American Psychiatric Association, 2000). Schizophrenia is one of the most disabling mental illnesses and it affects a person's personality, perception, cognition, emotion, and behaviors. Consequently, it causes disturbances to a person's social, interpersonal, and vocational functioning. Five subtypes of schizophrenia exist: paranoid type, disorganized type, catatonic type, undifferentiated type, and residual type.

It is estimated that three in 1,000 people suffer from schizophrenia in Hong Kong (Health and Welfare Bureau, 1999). Of the 14,480 total people suffering from schizophrenia, 70 percent need rehabilitation services. In fact, people with schizophrenia make up the majority of users of psychiatric rehabilitation services in Hong Kong, and they usually require a combination of medical, social, and vocational psychiatric rehabilitation services. Many attend outpatient clinics periodically and inpatient treatment occasionally, and some may require vocational rehabilitation services such as sheltered workshops and supported employment. Others may need residential services such as halfway houses and long-term care homes. Other supportive community services are available as well, such as community psychiatric treatment (CPT) teams and community psychiatric nurses (CPNs), that help persons with schizophrenia live as independently as possible in the community. The objectives of these services focus on *care* rather than cure and on *rehabilitation* rather than recovery.

ASSESSMENT

The vulnerability-stress model first outlined in Chapter 2 was originally developed for understanding, assessing, and treating people with schizophrenia (Yank, Bently, & Hargrove, 1993). This model emphasizes the interactive effect of biological, psychological, and social factors in determining the severity of mental illness. The following sections describe how this model can be used for treating schizophrenia.

Genetic Factors

Recent developments in understanding schizophrenia suggest that genetic/biological components play an important part in the etiology of schizophrenia. For example, studies have revealed that the concordant rate of the occurrence of schizophrenia among monozygotic twins is about 50 to 60 percent (Mueser & Gingerich, 1994). Moreover, it is rather common for individuals with schizophrenia to develop psychotic symptoms during adolescence. Although it is still unclear about the exact genetic mechanisms that lead to the development of schizophrenia, it has been found that people suffering from schizophrenia have a higher level of dopamine (a kind of neurotransmitter) than that of the general population. Simply put, people with schizophrenia emit a greater amount of dopamine than the corresponding receptors in the brain can accommodate, thus causing positive symptoms such as hallucinations (Mueser & Gingerich, 1994). However, it is still debatable as to whether the imbalance is a cause or a result of schizophrenia. However, it is generally agreed upon that positive symptoms are very disturbing to the client and affect his or her functioning. For example, a client of mine suffered from an auditory hallucination of a female voice telling him that he was good for nothing. The content of the voice was itself distressing, but the voice had become so frequent that my client became so distracted by it that he could not easily concentrate on and accomplish daily tasks.

It has also been suggested that this excessive dopamine level affects the cognitive functioning of an individual with schizophrenia (Yank et al., 1993). In essence, the person has difficulty processing incoming information, selecting the appropriate information, deriving plans of action, and carrying out action plans. As a result, the person is simply unable to respond and act appropriately in certain situations. For example, when a person with schizophrenia is confronted with different stimuli, he or she may become overwhelmed and unable to clearly differentiate the salient stimuli from the unimportant and is therefore unable to derive an action plan to deal with the situation. Coupled with the presence of active hallucinations or delusions, the person with schizophrenia may easily be overcome by ordinary circumstances and cannot perform such simple daily-living tasks as brushing his or her teeth. The high level of dopamine is said to create a lower stress threshold for clients with schizophrenia, making it more difficult for them to withstand stress and making them more vulnerable to developing schizophrenia.

Psychosocial Factors

It must be stated that simply because a person has a low stress threshold does not mean they will develop schizophrenia. On the other hand, it is certainly possible that an individual with a high stress threshold can develop schizophrenia. It all depends on the level of psychosocial stress encountered by the individual. In other words, regardless of whether it is high or low, when a person's stress level is above and beyond his or her particular stress threshold, he or she can develop schizophrenia. Since the trend is that a client with schizophrenia usually has a lower stress threshold, even a slight change in personal and psychosocial conditions can easily produce enough stress to cross his or her stress threshold and cause a relapse. An individual with schizophrenia is similar to an acrobat walking on a tight rope: both could fall to the ground easily should the breeze blow just so. As a worker, it is important to be sensitive to the client's changes in personal and psychosocial conditions and to assess his or her capacity to withstand those stresses. To conclude, this model can be presented in the following manner:

[Excessive dopamine secretion →
Presence of positive and negative symptoms ×
Cognitive dysfunction →
Lower stress threshold] + Environmental stress ×
Inadequate personal and environmental protectors → ·
Schizophrenia

AREAS OF ASSESSMENT
AND INTERVENTION

According to the vulnerability-stress model, four areas should be targeted for assessment and intervention: (1) medical and/or biochemical aspects, (2) personal protectors and risk factors, (3) environmental stressors, and (4) environmental protectors. Stress and protective factors that influence schizophrenia are presented in Table 6.1.

Medical and/or Biochemical Aspects

Medical Aspect

Family history of schizophrenia. It is important to obtain a detailed family medical history from the client and/or his or her relatives. As suggested, a strong genetic component may influence the development of schizophrenia among some clients. Indeed, it is not uncommon to find that some parents and siblings may also be suffering from schizophrenia. A client with a strong family history of schizophrenia may have a poorer diagnosis than a client without such a history, and therefore he or she may succumb more easily to psychosocial stress. Thus, a mental health worker must be very careful in making rehabili-

TABLE 6.1. Risk Factors and Protectors Influencing the Mental State of a Person with Schizophrenia

Factors	Biological	Psychological	Social
Risk factors	Positive symptoms—hallucinations, delusions Negative symptoms—lack of motivation, inadequate social and life skills	Cognitive malfunctions—poor problem-solving skills, poor judgment Adverse personal state	Stressful life changes High expressed emotions in the family Poor interpersonal relationships
Protectors	Compliant to medications	Good coping skills Personal strengths	Low expressed emotions in the family Good interpersonal relationships Availability of community services

tation plans with the client, outlining each step of the rehabilitation process and helping the individual gradually increase his or her stress threshold. Another important point is that the worker also needs to help the client and his or her family members make realistic expectations of rehabilitation outcomes. Generally, people with chronic schizophrenia may not or cannot make drastic and substantial improvement in social and occupational functioning.

History of illness and hospitalizations. It is necessary to obtain the history of the client's onset of illness, number of relapses, and numbers, circumstances, and reasons for admission to hospitals. Specifically, the worker needs to understand the client's severity of illness (e.g., involving self-harm or not), symptoms manifestations (e.g., types of hallucinations experienced), and circumstances leading to hospitalization or relapse (e.g., environmental stressors, drug compliance, and ways in which the client coped with the situations). This information is extremely useful for relapse prevention. In clinical practice, it is not uncommon to find that a client with schizophrenia follows a predictable pattern of relapse. As part of the relapse prevention strategy, this information can help the client and the worker identify the early signs of relapse and develop strategies to prevent it from happening.

Case example. Jerry was a thirty-two-year-old man with a fifteen-year history of schizophrenia. In that time, he had had four relapses and was admitted to the hospital each time. His relapse pattern included having very elevated moods, mentioning that he was the second son of God and that he was sent to save the world (grandiose delusion), refusing to take medications, and becoming more and more argumentative with family members. With this information the worker was able to help Jerry develop strategies to prevent another relapse.

Client's understanding and acceptance of illness. It is not uncommon to find that some clients with schizophrenia lack insight into their illness. They simply do not accept that they have schizophrenia and consequently refuse to take antipsychotic medications and decline to participate in rehabilitation programs. As a result, some experience further relapses. Clinical experiences suggest that a number of reasons exist for this lack of insight. First, some clients do not have adequate knowledge of schizophrenia and may also harbor incorrect information about the illness. For example, a client and his or her family may perceive schizophrenia as a personality deficit, and expect his or her mental state to improve with a change in personality (Wong & Poon, 2002). Another reason is related to social stigma. In Hong Kong, mental illness in general, and schizophrenia in particular, is heavily stigmatized (Hong Kong Council of Social Services & MHAHK, 1996, 1997). People with schizophrenia do not want to be labeled as such. The worker needs to explore this with his or her client and develop strategies to help the client accept their illness and ignore the associated stigma.

Primary or secondary diagnosis. It is useful to examine whether a client suffering from schizophrenia has another diagnosis such as depression or drug and alcohol dependence. Such a distinction may have implications for intervention. For example, a person suffering from a primary diagnosis of schizophrenia may also have depression. In this instance, depression may actually be a result of schizophrenia (e.g., feeling extremely disturbed by the voice), and is thus considered as a secondary illness. However, in the case of drug-induced psychosis, a person suffering from drug dependence may also have psychotic experiences. However, when the person abstains from taking the illicit drugs, he or she may not experience psychosis again. Thus, the drugs cause the psychosis and schizophrenia is seen as secondary to drug dependence. The treatment should then center on helping the client develop strategies to abstain from taking illicit drugs. Generally speaking, classifying an illness into primary or secondary categories helps to identify the major intervention focus. When the primary illness is successfully treated, the secondary illness will often be lifted.

Biochemical Factors

As mentioned, excessive dopamine secretion, which leads to the presence of positive symptoms and problems in information processing, is related to the development of schizophrenia. In the assessment it is important to explore the extent to which the positive and negative symptoms are affecting a client's social and occupational functioning. Since it is fairly common for a client with active psychotic symptoms to experience excessive emotions such as depressed moods or an elevated anxiety level (American Psychiatric Association, 2000), the worker needs to examine the emotional state of this client as well.

Positive symptoms. Hallucination involves an altered perceptual state (American Psychiatric Association, 2000). A client suffering hallucinations experiences distortions in any of the five senses: vision, hearing, smell, touch, and taste. Auditory hallucination is the most common type of hallucinatory experience found in persons with schizophrenia. Examples include hearing critical voices; a woman seeing a cross turning in her head; constantly smelling bad odor; feeling bugs crawling on one's body; and vomiting from a percieved bad taste. Individuals with schizophrenia may experience a predictable pattern of hallucinations during the active phase, residual phase, and relapses. It is useful for the worker to get a history of the client's pattern of hallucination and to monitor his or her mental state by inquiring about the degree of insight and self-mastery of these hallucinations. A client is said to be mentally unwell when he or she makes more complaints about the hallucinations, finds the hallucinations becoming more and more unbearable, and begins to follow the instructions of the voices and/or reacts strongly against the hallucinations.

Delusions are erroneous and fixed beliefs that usually involve a misinterpretation of perceptions or experiences. These may include persecutory ideas (e.g., people in the street are after me); grandiose ideas (e.g., I am all powerful and responsible for everything, good or bad); ideas of reference (e.g., that people in the radio/TV are talking about me); and religious beliefs (e.g., God punishes me by asking me to sit in a chair for days). The most common types of delusions are persecutory ideas and delusions of reference. Some people with schizophrenia may develop a persecutory delusional system. These individuals gradually include more and more people into a delusional system, claiming that these individuals conspire to persecute them. For example, a resident in a halfway house complained that his roommate harassed him and always played tricks on him. Gradually, he felt that other roommates were having the same attitude toward him. When the worker intervened, the client even started to think that the worker was siding with the other roommates. In the end, almost everyone in the halfway house was acting against him.

Abnormal thought processes include psychotic features such as thought broadcast (believing that everyone knows what he or she is thinking), thought block (cannot think of anything; the mind is blank), and thought insertion (thinking that outside thoughts are inserted into his or her mind).

Since a client may perform bizarre and aggressive behaviors when he or she is under psychotic influences, the worker needs to assess the client's *level of reality contact*. Essentially, a person with poor reality contact may respond in words and/or actions toward his or her hallucinations and delusions. For example, a worker may ask the client: "Since you believe that he is trying to kill you, what do you think you will do?" By asking this and similar questions, the worker can gauge the severity of the client's psychotic experience and the extent to which he or she will react. In the residual phase, despite medications, a client may still experience positive symptoms, but with much reality contact. In other words, the client is able to distinguish, to some extent, that the hallucinations or delusions are unreal and can derive some strategies to deal with the hallucinations and delusions.

A client's level of reality contact can be detected in two ways: (1) the client is more inclined to act upon the influence of the positive symptoms and (2) due to preoccupation with the symptoms, the client shows gradual or marked deterioration in social and occupational functioning. Since clients with chronic schizophrenia still experience psychotic symptoms in the residual phase, they are assessed to be mentally unstable when the two factors are present.

Negative symptoms. Negative symptoms are characterized by the presence of the following symptoms in a person with schizophrenia: flattened affect, inability to experience feelings, lack of motivation or volition, poverty of speech, social withdrawal, and neglect of self-care (Mueser & Gingerich, 1994). This set of symptoms can be as damaging to the functioning of the clients as the positive symptoms. Clients with prominent negative symptoms usually lack motivation to participate in the various rehabilitation services, and the worker needs to put a great deal of effort into engaging the clients in the rehabilitation process. Moreover, these individuals lack many skills, ranging from basic self-care skills to interpersonal skills, social skills, domestic-living skills, etc. Therefore, it is very common for these individuals with prominent negative symptoms to undergo skills training during their rehabilitation process.

One of the thorny issues regarding negative symptoms is the lack of motivation found among some clients with schizophrenia. Mental health workers often complain that their clients lack motivation and cannot be easily encouraged to engage in the rehabilitation process. Although each client is unique, a few common reasons are often mentioned for such a lack of motivation. First, some antipsychotic medications have sedative effects, and those clients who are on a heavy dosage may become lethargic and lack energy. Sometimes, if possible, a change in medication may reduce such side effects. Also, an alteration in the schedule of the intake of medication may be useful to reduce the sedative effects of medication for some clients. For example, if a person feels very tired and has difficulty getting up in the morning after taking medication, it is possible for him or her to take the medicine a bit earlier in the evening so that the effects of medication are not as strong in the morning. However, a reduction or a change in the schedule of medications may result in a relative increase in the client's positive symptoms. The mental health worker needs to work closely with the psychiatrist and client to establish the client's appropriate minimum dosage.

Adverse personal reaction to schizophrenia may also affect the motivation of the client by hampering his or her self-esteem and confidence. Clients who have lost their ability to do their normal activities and are socially disadvantaged and can easily develop low self-esteem. Others may have acquired a sick role and a sense of dependency on the mental health care system (Mueser & Gingerich, 1994). Under these circumstances, one of the major rehabilitation goals is to help these individuals acquire positive experiences so that they can rebuild or strengthen their self-esteem and confidence. The strengths model of rehabilitation can serve as a guiding intervention model for enhancing the motivation of some clients with poor volition (see Chapter 3).

Cognitive malfunctions. As previously mentioned, an excessive dopamine level affects the cognitive functioning of an individual with schizophrenia. In essence, the person is unable to engage in the process of receiving information, discriminating the appropriate information from the inappropriate, deriving plans of action, and carrying out an action plan. The person is simply unable to respond and act appropriately to daily situations. These cognitive deficits may result in a number of problems faced by a person with schizophrenia, such as poor concentration and impaired judgment, poor response time, and poor problem-solving and coping abilities. Moreover, it may also be difficult for him or her to engage in complex and abstract thinking and the person often benefits from concrete, simple, and short conversations. Indeed, it is more effective to use behavioral and skills training approaches in working with a client with severe cognitive impairments.

Understanding Client's Medical Treatment

Effects and side effects of medication. It is important for the worker to know the type of antipsychotic medication his or her client is taking and its proper effects. The worker should always ask the client for this information, and should educate him or her on the effects and side effects of the medication, inform the medical staff of any possible adverse effects due to a change in medications, and discuss with doctors a reduction or increase in medications when change in a client's mental state occurs. The worker may also need to help the client find ways to manage the side effects of medications. Some side effects are quite disturbing to the client, and he or she must know of and be prepared for them. The worker should also work closely with the psychiatrist to implement a possible change in medications should the side effects become too severe for the clients.

Client's understanding and compliance to medications. Since medication is an important protective factor against a client's relapse, it is always helpful to get a sense of whether he or she is compliant to medications. If he or she is not compliant, he or she may have a greater chance of relapse (Marder, 1986). Several possible reasons exist for the client's lack of compliance with medications. First, some clients find the side effects of medications intolerable and therefore refuse to take the medication. Others do not have adequate knowledge of the effects and side effects of medications and harbor some misunderstanding, and for this reason decline to take the medicines. For example, a client of mine believed that the medications he was taking was the reason for to his sexual impotence (his psychiatrist did not agree), and another client said that the medication was strong and upset her bodily internal balance, causing her to experience a variety of physical discomforts. In any case, clients may have an idiosyncratic understanding (i.e., misunderstanding) of the effects and side effects of medications and consequently refuse to take them.

Besides the issues of knowledge and understanding of medications, the lack of compliance with medications may also be related to the social stigma attached to schizophrenia. As mentioned, schizophrenia is heavily stigmatized in Hong Kong. Some clients reject the label and refuse to take the medications. Clients often want to know how they can hide their mental illness from their co-workers, particularly in relation to taking medications and regular psychiatric follow-ups. In fact, some clients who do not discuss this issue with their mental health workers may simply stop taking the medications when they are confronted with these situations. Understanding a client's reasons for noncompliance can help the worker facilitate the client in developing practical strategies to overcome the problems.

Alternative medicines. Some clients with schizophrenia in Hong Kong may take alternative Chinese medicines in addition to Western medicine. The worker in this instance should advise the client to be cautious of any unhealthy side effects of mixing the two types of medicines together. Family members and clients are often quite willing to discuss this issue, and the worker should encourage them to seek further advice from their psychiatrists.

Interventions in the Medical/Biochemical Aspects

Medications. A study revealed that about 70 percent of people in the United States suffering from schizophrenia who did not take medications experienced a psychotic relapse within one year after hospitalization. However, only 30 percent of those who complied with medication experienced a psychotic relapse (Mueser & Gingerich, 1994). This study supports the notion that medication is necessary, although not wholly sufficient to stablize a client's mental state.

The typical antipsychotics (neuroleptics) include haloperidol, chlorpromazine, and thioridazine. Most are given as tablets or syrup. Some (e.g., zuclopenthixol, flupenthixol) are available as long-lasting (two to six weeks) depot injections (Marder, 1986). Unfortunately, these typical antipsychotics have a range of side effects, such as severe movement disorders, called extrapyramidal side effects. These include muscle spasms, unusual body movements, involuntary movement disorders such as limb rigidity and tremor, and tardive dyskinesia (unusual and repetitive movements of the body, especially of the face, tongue, and neck muscles) (Marder, 1986). Extrapyramidal side effects are perhaps the most difficult side effects with which to live.

Atypical antipsychotics are a relatively recent development in medication for people with schizophrenia and other psychotic illnesses. These atypical antipsychotics include clozapine, risperidone, olanzapine, and quetiapine (Marder, 1986). Their side effects are believed to be milder than typical antipsychotics, but they are more expensive. In some countries, such as the United States, atypical antipsychotics comprise 80 percent of antipsychotic medication prescriptions, but in Hong Kong only a small percentage of the persons with schizophrenia are given these new medications. The most commonly prescribed atypical antipsychotics are risperidone and olanzapine. Clozapine is particularly effective for people who have failed to respond to other drugs, but is usually given as a last resort. This is because it is linked to a rare but potentially lethal side effect—white blood cell disruption (Marder, 1986). Side effects of atypical antipsychotics include weight gain, drowsiness, rapid heartbeat, and dizziness when changing position.

Education. At present, medications are still a crucial part of treatment for schizophrenia. Since many clients do not have an adequate understanding of the effects and side effects of antipsychotics, the worker needs to have sufficient knowledge of these effects and be able to educate the clients on which medications can best help them control their positive symptoms and raise their stress threshold. It is hoped that by increasing the client's knowledge of the medications, he or she will be more accepting and compliant to them. It is often useful to introduce the concept of *minimum therapeutic dosage* to a client. He or she must know both the benefits and the side effects of the antipsychotics, and should take only the minimum dosage necessary for the medication to be effective. Moreover, this concept also supports an increase or a decrease in medications at different times in a client's life (depending on his or her level of stress). In other words, while the client is maintained on a minimum therapeutic dosage, the worker may negotiate with the psychiatrist to increase or decrease medication during times of distress or stability. The advantage of introducing this concept of minimum dosage to the client is that it provides him or her with more control over the intake of medications and his or her rehabilitation process. Indeed, the client needs to have a greater understanding of his or her personal conditions and should help plan and decide the level of medications he or she needs.

The worker should also ask if the mental state of the client is controllable under medication. If the client is experiencing an active psychotic state, it is necessary to examine whether he or she needs hospitalization or if an adjustment in the dosage of medication would be sufficient to maintain stability.

Strategies for handling positive and negative symptoms. It is necessary for the worker to appreciate the agonies and fear that accompany a client's experience of positive symptoms. To the client, the experiences are real and produce a gamut of negative emotions. Moreover, under these psychotic influences, a client may perform bizarre and aggressive behaviors about which he or she may feel very embarrassed afterward. During the active and acute episode, it is advisable for the worker to do the following:

- Empathize with the client's feelings associated with the delusions and hallucinations. (Let the client know that his or her feelings are understood.)
- Do not argue with the client about his or her hallucinations and delusions. In fact, the more a worker tries to argue with the client, the more avowed his or her delusions or hallucinations may become. This point is particularly valid for people with delusions. It is important for the worker to keep in mind that offering the client support does not mean confirming his or her hallucinations or delusions. The worker should support the client by only empathizing with the client's feelings associated with the delusions or hallucinations. For example, a worker may say, "You seem rather agitated and distressed by the voices. Is there something you can do to make yourself feel a bit better when you hear the voices?" This addresses the emotions, not the content of the voice.
- Help the client and family members make realistic expectations of the rehabilitation outcomes. This is not easy for a client with a relatively short history of illness. The worker needs to help him or her and the family members accept that the client's functioning level may not be the same as what it was before the illness. For example, a client of mine, after college graduation, believed he could engage in higher-paying office work. His parents thought the same. However, he had prominent negative symptoms and could not maintain stability in such a stressful situation. After a few trials and much disappointment, he began to accept the limitations posed by his ill-

ness. Eventually, he accepted a job as a messenger. Thus, it is important to help the client and the family members make realistic rehabilitation plans. Indeed, the worker and the client must constantly assess the level of stress the client can handle during certain periods of his or her life. It is necessary for the worker to bear in mind the concept of walking on a tightrope. The worker has to help the client strike a balance between what he or she wants to achieve and what his or her health conditions allow. It is recommended that the worker adopt an incremental, step-by-step approach for the client's rehabilitation goals. Rehabilitation goals should be broken down into small, achievable steps, and should be carefully staged so that the client can gradually build up the skills and confidence necessary to fulfill the tasks.

- Engage the client in concrete and behavioral tasks, not in abstract tasks. Since a client with schizophrenia may have severe cognitive dysfunctions it is necessary for the worker to avoid designing complex learning tasks and to simplify and break down learning goals into concrete, behavioral tasks. Likewise, the worker should speak to the client in simple, short, and concise sentences.
- Teach coping skills for handling positive and negative symptoms. Many clients still have positive and negative symptoms even when taking medication. The worker and the client should discuss ways of managing these symptoms. For example, a client of mine had serious residual auditory hallucination and felt rather annoyed by the voices, particularly when she was sitting in the bus. I encouraged her to buy a pocket-size radio and listen to radio programs when traveling on the bus. This turned out to be a workable solution. Successful coping skills are concrete, simple, and behavioral, and can be performed easily to cope with the situationally specific symptoms. These coping skills should be derived in consultation with the client. It is always helpful for the worker to countercheck with the client about the effectiveness of the coping skills. For example, "On the scale of 10, with 0 being ineffective and 10 being very effective, how would you rate the coping skill?"
- Encourage the client to engage in activities to minimize negative symptoms. This is especially important for people with chronic schizophrenia. Although individuals still may not participate actively in rehabilitation programs, the structures of such programs can help them to be less withdrawn. In Hong Kong, day activity

centers and social clubs are examples of the day programs available for people with chronic mental illness.

Personal Protectors and Risk Factors

A number of factors are subsumed under this heading. These include: (1) adverse psychological state, (2) skills deficits, (3) personal strength.

Adverse Psychological State

During the course of rehabilitation, some clients with schizophrenia develop very low self-esteem. A number of reasons may account for this. First, due to psychiatric impairments, these clients may experience a great number of losses, such as jobs, friends, financial security, and above all, personhood. It is not uncommon for these individuals to feel that they are no longer the persons they used to be and that people treat them as if they are of a marginal status in the society. Second, persons with psychiatric illnesses, particularly schizophrenia, are highly stigmatized in society. This stigma causes them to be socially disadvantaged and they may be discriminated against in social and occupational roles. Therefore, it is not surprising to find that people with schizophrenia may gradually acquire a negative view of themselves. A vicious cycle occurs when these individuals with low self-esteem begin to feel apathetic and powerless. As soon as they resign to a state of hopelessness they give up on themselves and refuse to participate in the rehabilitation process. It is not uncommon to find people with chronic schizophrenia to have acquired such a hopeless and powerless state. Thus, the worker needs to assess whether and to what extent his or her client has developed this adverse psychological state.

Skills Deficits

Skills deficits is another important area for assessment. As mentioned, due to cognitive dysfunctions, some people with schizophrenia have suffered from a certain degree of skills deficits, some more serious than others. Poor performance in requisite and functional skills may have far-reaching consequences on a client's independent and community living. A thorough assessment in skill performance is necessary so that skills training can be arranged for the client to facilitate the acquisitions of social skills and independent-living skills.

Skills for social role performance. This set of skills is generically called social skills (Vaccaro, Pitts, & Wallace, 1992), and is necessary for satisfactory performance in roles such as friend, family member, worker, and partner. A client's inability to perform adequately in any of these social roles can create a great deal of stress for him or her. Moreover, successful performances in these roles can lead to other benefits, such as having more social support from others. Generally, these skills can be further broken down into receiving skills (e.g., appropriately nodding one's head), sending skills (e.g., tone of voice), and processing skills (e.g., focusing on relevant information in a conversation). Each role may have a specific set of receiving, sending, and processing skills, therefore, the worker needs to assess these skills under specific role conditions. For example, specific skills must be learned when a client becomes a father.

Skills for independent living. This is another set of skills that many of our clients with chronic schizophrenia need to learn in order to live independently in a community. These skills concern self-care, domestic-living, health maintenance, leisure, transportation, and money management. It is not uncommon for the worker to use a checklist approach to assess a client's overall level of performance in the previously mentioned skill areas. In the assessment, the worker has to clearly identify the client's areas of skills deficits.

Personal Strength

The worker should examine the strengths of the client as well. Instead of focusing only on a client's deficits and problems, the worker should look closely into the client's desires, goals, ambitions, and hopes, and should develop his or her internal and external resources to fulfill his or her goals. The ultimate objective is for the client to use his or her own internal and external resources to achieve his or her own rehabilitation goals. It is paramount to note that the client must be actively involved in the process of change. The client should make as many decisions as he or she is capable of making, and should see that these decisions and actions do affect his or her well-being. The worker needs to assess the client's internal resources such as aspirations and competencies and external resources such as material resources, and the worker should also assess the client's support network.

Interventions

Empathize with the client's psychological pains and reactions to having schizophrenia. Since some clients may develop an adverse psychological state as a result of developing schizophrenia, the worker needs to empathize with the pain and losses the client is experiencing. It is sometimes difficult to fully understand clients' experiences. Indeed, unless one is personally experiencing positive symptoms, negative symptoms, and delusional thoughts because of schizophrenia, one cannot fully comprehend the depth of the pain, agony, loss, etc., associated with the disease. Regardless, the worker can openly acknowledge a client's struggle by understanding and helping the client manage his or her experiences. It is important for the worker to acknowledge and not deny the client's experiences. Skills such as empathy, genuineness, and unconditional positive regard are useful for working with people with schizophrenia.

Supportive counseling. This is a term that is often used to describe the nature of counseling provided to persons with schizophrenia. Torrey (1988) suggests that supportive therapy

> provides a patient with friendship, encouragement, practical advice such as access to community resources or how to develop a more active social life, vocational counselling, suggestions for minimizing friction with family members, and, above all, hope that the person's life may be improved. Discussions focus on the here-and-now, not the past, and on problems of living encountered by the patient as he or she tries to meet the exigencies of life, despite a handicapping brain disease. (Torrey, 1988, p. 259)

It is to be distinguished from insight-oriented psychotherapy—the uncovering and exploration of unconscious conflicts. He notes that "insight-oriented psychotherapy is of no value for people with schizophrenia" (Torrey, 1988, p. 220). However, Torrey (1988) further explains that this comment does not mean that the person with schizophrenia, as any other person, cannot benefit from understanding himself or herself better. The emphasis against insight-oriented therapy is because the impairments of people with schizophrenia tend to be psychiatric, including cognitive dysfunctions, and therefore it is more useful to provide practical advice and assistance so that these individuals can develop life skills such as managing medication, learning to socialize, handling finances, and getting a job. Moreover, these individuals also can benefit from emotional support when going through their illness. Support can help them through difficult times and ease their feeling of isolation.

Supportive counseling incorporates a strengths focus. Throughout the rehabilitation process, the worker should explore the client's resources for fulfilling his or her own rehabilitation goals. Although it is necessary to help the client identify goals, it is more important for the client to make decisions throughout the process of formulating and achieving goals. The worker should bear in mind two important underlying principles. First, the worker should help the client gain successful experiences and view negative experiences in a positive and balanced light. Second, the worker must help the client to understand that he or she has contributed greatly to the successful experiences. The ultimate objective is to empower the client by showing him or her what he or she has done that resulted in personal success.

Skills training for persons with schizophrenia. Skills training generally adopts a behavioral approach in the intervention process.

Case example. Mr. Choy was living in a halfway house and was identified as having self-care problems. Residents of the house often complained of his body smell. Because of this and for possible health reasons, staff of a sheltered workshop were reluctant to accept him into the workshop.

The worker helped Mr. Choy identify and specify the target behaviors. It was found that Mr. Choy had the following skills problems:

- did not comb his hair (skills deficit)
- did not wash himself (skills deficit)
- spit on the floor in the house and at work (inappropriate behaviors)
- did not trim his nails, and the nails were very dirty (skills deficit)
- did not change and wash his clothes, including underwear (skills deficit)

His key worker in the halfway house was asked to conduct a one-week assessment of his skill problems and to establish a baseline for each problem. The worker observed and discussed with Mr. Choy reasons why he could not perform these skills (maintenance factors—factors that reinforce certain behaviors to occur or not occur), as well as the activities he liked and disliked (reinforcers) (Martin & Pear, 1999). It was realized that Mr. Choy had been living alone and away from others for so long that he had forgotten or had never developed the habits of regular self-care. Moreover, he had no incentive or disincentive to perform the necessary self-care skills while he was living on his own.

A token system was chosen to help Mr. Choy develop self-care skills. The key worker and Mr. Choy negotiated the specific goals to be achieved weekly (e.g., taking showers on alternate nights initially, since he refused to do it every day) and the ways in which the token system operated (e.g., ten points for reaching each goal with prizes earned by these points, such as a can of soda for fifty points and a movie ticket for two hundred). Mr. Choy made several suggestions for the token system which were eventually adopted. They both agreed to review the progress weekly. With time, the actual physical rewards were replaced by social reinforcements.

Besides independent-living skills, some people with schizophrenia need training in social skills as well. The following case example outlines this need.

Mr. Cheung was a twenty-one-year-old man with a five-year history of schizophrenia. It did not take long for anyone to notice that Mr. Cheung had very poor social skills. He spoke with a loud voice (almost shouting), and would interrupt a conversation whenever he wanted to speak. He made very little eye contact and stood very close to others. He came to my office one day and said he was very frustrated that people did not want to befriend him. He did not know why people reacted to him in such negative ways. Since I had known him for a short while, I asked if he knew that his social skills might be the culprits. He acknowledged that some people had mentioned so, but did not know what was wrong with his social skills. I invited him to ask his friends to permit him to videotape a half hour conversation with them. In the next meeting, we analyzed the conversation and pointed out the problems in his sending and receiving skills. Specifically, in terms his sending skills, he shouted instead of speaking. He spoke very quickly as well, interrupting conversation at the wrong time. As for his receiving skills, he lacked appropriate eye contact and social distance. During the next few sessions I practiced sending and receiving skills with him. I then asked him to invite another friend to the session and videotaped their conversations. We then watched this recording and identified the problem areas. For each problem identified, I asked Mr. Cheung to practice the skills until he fully acquired them. Since Mr. Cheung was the type who did not benefit strictly from "talk" therapy, this practical-skill training approach was very effective.

Environmental Stressors

Changing Life Circumstances

As mentioned before, people suffering from schizophrenia are more susceptible to stress because they often have a lower stress threshold than the general population. Therefore, slight changes in a person's life can become very stressful and critical and can adversely affect his or her mental state. Examples of these changes are a transition from the hospital back to the community, starting a new job, entering a new relationship, etc. During such critical periods an individual with schizophrenia may experience more symptoms and is more vulnerable to relapse. Therefore, during the periodic assessment of a client's mental state the worker needs to identify whether any change has occurred or will occur in the client's life circumstances and assess what the client needs in order to successfully manage the change.

Patterns of Environmental Stress and Coping

Another aspect of assessment is to examine if the client is particularly vulnerable to relapse under certain environmental stressors. The worker needs to obtain a history of the types of environmental stressors associated with a client's previous relapses and ways in which the client tried to cope with the stress. If a certain pattern is detected, the worker can help the client learn ways of handling such environmental stress in the future, encourage the client to avoid encountering this stressful environmental condition, and help the client modify the stressful environment. For example, I had a client who often experienced relapses when she started looking for open employment. Particularly, she found the interviews rather stressful. She claimed she did not know how and what to talk about and was afraid that they knew of her illness. We then discussed and developed strategies to overcome these stressful circumstances.

Family Climate

Family climate is another important environmental stressor that should be assessed thoroughly by the worker. Since this is discussed in detail in Chapter 8, this section will present only the basic concepts of family climate. According to Leff and Vaughn (1981), certain family attitudes, termed high expressed emotions (HEE), are associated with a higher relapse rate found in persons with schizophrenia. They revealed that clients living with family members who exhibit critical comments, hostility, and overinvolvement (doing everything for the client, being overprotective, etc.) had a higher rate of relapse than those with family members without these attitudes. The rates of relapse for HEE was 44 percent and for LEE (low expressed emotion) families was 5 percent (Falloon, Boyd, McGill, Strang, & Moss, 1981). Thus, it is important to assess whether the atmosphere in a client's family contains these attitudes. If HEE are present, the worker must either work with the family members to reduce these habits or provide an alternative accommodation for the client if these attitudes cannot be adequately modified.

Intervention

Help the client to understand the impact of stress on his or her mental state. Some clients may not be aware of the detrimental effects of stress on their mental conditions. It is important for the worker to educate his or her client about the vulnerability-stress concept in simple, everyday language. For example, "Some people are born less resistant to stress than others, and as a result they may develop mental health problems. As well, people with schizophrenia are born with excessive chemical substances in their brains that prevent it from coping with stress, allowing a breakdown even with a relatively small amount of stress. It is similar to diabetics who are born with too much sugar in their bodies for whom a small intake of sugar can upset their internal bodily balance." When the client begins to accept this idea, the worker can go through the client's history of relapse and identify the pattern of psychosocial stresses that affected him or her in the past. The worker also needs to discuss what coping skills the client should use to handle these psychosocial stresses.

Gradually expose clients to stressful social environments. Some stressful social situations are unavoidable, and clients are bound to face these situations at some point in their lives. If the stressful situations are identified, the worker can help the clients gradually approach them. I had a client who felt particularly stressed whenever he had to face his stepfather. He went home every weekend and would have dinner with his mother and that stepfather. His returns to the halfway house on Mondays were characterized by excessive anger, agitation, and argument. On a few occasions he showed signs of relapse. I discussed with him his encounters at home and how he perceived his stepfather. I also helped him develop some coping strategies to help manage his emotions during and after the encounters.

Monitor the client's mental state closely during times of stress. The worker should take special note and offer extra support when he or she recognizes that his or her client is undergoing stressful life circumstances. This may be in the forms of home visits, coping-skills training, and negotiation with the client's psychiatrist to increase medication. Indeed, the worker needs to communicate very closely with the client, with the client's psychiatrist, and with the related mental health service providers during this critical period. These parties must work out a plan as to whether medications need to be adjusted, exposure to certain psychosocial stress needs to be reduced, and whether the level of support to the client needs to be increased.

Reduce the negative family climate. Falloon et al. (1988) have developed specific family therapies to address the HEE among family members. Results have been positive. Details of these family therapies are discussed in Chapter 8.

Environmental Protectors

Protective buffers to stress are available for persons with schizophrenia. It is important for the worker to identify and assess these areas and find ways to strengthen or build these environmental protectors. The protectors to be identified are availability of community rehabilitation services, friendship support network, and family support network. However, the worker needs to be aware that any protector can also be a potential risk factor, and that each of these factors may have a different meaning for each individual.

Availability of Community Rehabilitation Services

Generally speaking, people with schizophrenia who are supported by the community rehabilitation services achieve better social functioning and fewer hospitalizations than those who do not receive adequate supportive community rehabilitation services (Mueser & Gingerich, 1994). Several reasons may be ascribed to such positive results. First, services that contain meaningful daytime activities can help the client counteract his or her apathy and avolition resulting from being idle at home. Second, personnel working in these services form a formal support network for the client. Thus, when some clients are under stress they receive support from the staff. Some clients heavily rely on staff of various rehabilitation services such as halfway houses and sheltered workshops for social support. In assessment, the worker needs to examine whether his or her client will benefit from referrals to any community rehabilitation services or will be overwhelmed by such referrals and possible changes.

Friendship Support Network

A good friend can help an individual sail through difficult and stressful times. This certainly applies to people with schizophrenia. A worker should attempt to link up clients with one another (Walsh, 2000). This is done with the hope that they can form a support system. When the worker facilitates a client's move to independent community living, he or she should certainly explore whether the client has an identifiable support network. Sometimes the worker deliberately pairs up an individual client with another client so that they can provide support for each other in the community.

Family Support Network

Family members are among the most important providers of support for clients. Culturally speaking, family support is important for both family members and the client. This is because some family members feel no responsibility for their mentally ill relative, or they feel shame and guilt for being unable to take care of the disabled members (Wong, 2000). Family support also provides a client with a sense of familial love and lessens his or her feeling of abandonment. Furthermore, positive communication such as warmth and positive regard lead to better social functioning (Wong & Poon, 2002). However, as mentioned previously, family members can also be a stress factor for the client. It is important for the worker to assess the positive and negative impacts of family involvement on the well-being of the clients.

Interventions

Refer clients to community rehabilitation services. An important case management activity is for the worker to link his or her clients to community rehabilitation services. During the process, the worker must have the following skills:

- *Relationship and negotiation skills:* The worker needs to be able to develop adequate working relationships with a client and the personnel of the mental health system. The worker must negotiate the most appropriate services for the client. Clinical experience suggests that successful referrals not only depend on the availability of the services but also require the establishment of a good relationship between the worker and the personnel of other services.
- *Ability to follow up:* It is important for the worker to actively follow up on the initial referral to ensure that the client is receiving the required services. The worker needs to provide the personnel with adequate information about the client, and may have to negotiate with the personnel of other caregiving services so that the client can better adjust to a new environment. In addition, the worker may need to support the client during the initial period of change so that he or she can better adjust to the environment.
- *Advocacy:* It is not uncommon for a worker to encounter situations whereby, due to very rigid rules and regulations, the client's application for services is rejected. Sometimes a client does not receive the services because of the differences in assessment and clinical judgment between the personnel of the outside service units and the worker. In this circumstance, the worker needs to advocate the client's need of services, work out the differences, and find ways to fulfill the rules and regulations.

Help clients develop informal support networks. This is another direction in strengthening the environmental protective factor for the clients. The worker can use a number of strategies to develop a support network.

- *Mutual-aid groups:* Workers may link the clients to any mutual-aid groups so that they can find someone who shares their experiences. This also reduces clients' sense of isolation.

- *Buddy system:* Formal or informal opportunities should be provided for clients to develop close and supportive relationships. This should be done particularly for clients with weak family and friendship ties in the community. This system is useful for preparing clients with the intention of living together after moving out of the halfway house. Regardless of the setting, this is a useful strategy to help a client establish supportive friendship networks in the community.
- *Mentors.* Another popular way to involve clients in the community is to link them to a volunteer mentor. The ideal scenario is for a volunteer to see the client on a regular basis involving social activities. These activities can be friendly visits, shopping, going to the movies, etc. This type of volunteer programs is quite successfully run in the United States (e.g., Chinman, Weingarten, Stayner, & Davidson, 2001). However, a few difficulties occur in running these programs. First, it is hard to find volunteers who can regularly participate. Second, the workers need to provide a great amount of support for the volunteers. These factors notwithstanding, this is a good way of creating community spirit and providing friendship and mutual help.

Encourage family members to provide support. This will be discussed in greater detail in Chapter 8. It is worth mentioning here that family members are potential and or actual resources for the clients, and workers need to help members develop resources and provide ongoing support to fulfill their caring roles. Family members should not be left without support in their caregiving. Indeed, many studies have found that families experience a great deal of burdens and stress when coping with a mental illness (Wong, 2000).

GUIDELINES FOR WORKING WITH PERSONS WITH SCHIZOPHRENIA

Care versus Cure

Schizophrenia is a disabling mental illness that can be degenerative. Therefore, assessment and intervention focus on rehabilitation and care, not on cure.

Strengths versus Deficits

It is important to assess both deficits and strengths of the clients. Traditional approaches center too heavily on improving clients' deficits and ignore clients' strengths.

Supportive and Behavior-Oriented Counseling versus Insight-Oriented Counseling

The focus of assessment and intervention for treatment of schizophrenia should center on the functional issues essential for community living. The role of the worker is to support the clients along their pathway to rehabilitation. This is very different from some traditional psychotherapies that are insight oriented. Indeed, since clients have cognitive deficits, in-depth and insight-oriented psychotherapy must be used carefully for clients with schizophrenia. In general, the dominant approach for working with people suffering from schizophrenia is supportive and behavior-oriented counseling approaches.

Assertive Approach

An assertive approach has been empirically identified as an important element in community rehabilitation services (Test & Stein, 2000). It is important for workers to reach out to clients with schizophrenia. Moreover, workers need to actively link clients to formal and informal networks and services in the community.

Continuous Support

It is necessary to render ongoing support to clients so that they can be maintained in the community. Since the mental health conditions of persons with schizophrenia fluctuate over time, it is important to provide them with continuous support and to consistently monitor their mental state.

RELAPSE PREVENTION

Reasons for Relapse Prevention

Generally speaking, the more relapses a person experiences the poorer the prognosis, and the more chronic his or her conditions become (Mueser & Gingerich, 1994). Therefore, it is common for a worker to help a client develop a relapse prevention plan at some stage in his or her rehabilitation process. Early detection of relapse may prevent a person from hospitalization and thus reduce the cost of hospitalization. Early detection can also reduce personal and social costs. For instance, both the client and his or her family members may be saved from the trauma of having to go through the disorganization, anxiety, and anguish of a relapse.

Worker's Tasks in Relapse Prevention

Understand the Patterns of a Client's Relapse

As mentioned before, the worker should have a clear picture of the client's history of relapse or first episode of illness. Information to be sought includes: symptoms during prodromal phase, coping skills used by the client, and circumstances preceding a relapse, such as stressors and medication compliance.

Educate the Client and Family Members on the Client's Relapse Patterns

This is especially applicable to the client who is staying or expected to stay with his or her family members. The idea is to help the client and family members take note of a possible relapse.

Develop Action Plans

The worker can help the client and family develop an action plan once a possible relapse is detected. The plan should include specific strategies that each person is to do at a given moment. These strategies should be feasible and easily performed by the individuals.

Closely Monitor a Client's Mental State

A worker needs to closely monitor a client's mental state during the prodromal phase. He or she should help the client and family to make decisions about actions to be taken. Since relapse is a time of crisis, the worker must be directive and active in providing ideas and advice. However, it should be up to the client and the family to make the final decisions. In the case of possible harm to self or others, the worker may have to facilitate the process of admitting an involuntary client to the hospital.

Provide Immediate and Active Support During the Prodromal Phase

The prodromal phase is often a time of intense emotions during which the worker needs to provide support for the client and the family members. Confusion, anxiety, and indecision are some of the emotions facing the client and the family members during this period. It is timely for the worker to provide support for the family, and is also an opportunity for the worker to build a rapport with the family as well.

Negotiate with Personnel of Medical and Social Rehabilitation Services

During the time of relapse, the worker may need to solicit support from other services and mental health workers such as CPT teams, psychiatrists, social workers, etc. Clients and family members who are in a state of confusion may have to rely on the worker to make the liaison. Thus, the worker must be prepared to be active in the process.

CASE ILLUSTRATION

Mr. Hing was a twenty-four-year-old man suffering from schizophrenia. He developed the illness when he was nineteen and experienced auditory hallucinations of a woman's voice calling him "a good-for-nothing pig." He used to live with his family in public housing before he was referred to our halfway house. At home, he lived with his parents and two unmarried sisters. He had been working at a sheltered workshop for about four years.

Medical and/or Biochemical Aspects

Mr. Hing's immediate family had no history of schizophrenia. However, his maternal grandmother and one of his distant cousins had developed schizophrenia. As mentioned, the onset of his schizophrenia was at age nineteen, when he heard a woman's voice calling him "a good-for-nothing pig." He also felt that people knew what he was thinking (thought broadcast) and that they laughed at his silly thoughts.

Mr. Hing had experienced four relapses in the past five years. Each relapse was preceded by an increase in the frequency of the voice and the feeling of distress and agitation. When he lost contact with reality, he responded to the voice by disagreeing with it. On one occasion he even tried to commit suicide. When I asked him how he had tried to cope with the voice he could not offer any answer. It was his sisters who eventually brought him to the psychiatrist. He experienced thought broadcast only during the time of the onset of the illness, and did not experience it during relapses. He told me that he stopped taking the medication a month or so prior to his relapses. Moreover, he became more and more unhappy and frustrated at working in the sheltered workshop, thinking that he could do much better than being put in a place alongside the "dumb" people.

He was put on chlorpromazine, 400 mg daily, as well as trihexyphenidy. Depot medication was also given to Mr. Hing every four weeks. Besides suffering from the usual side effects of dry mouth and the feeling of restlessness, he had developed neuroleptic malignant syndrome, with the obvious sign of a wry neck (head permanently twisted to the left). This not only seriously affected his self-image, it also gave the family and Mr. Hing the wrong perception that psychotropic medication was toxic. Indeed, the family tried very hard to seek alternative medicines for Mr. Hing, and they discouraged him from taking the antipsychotic medications. Of course, Mr. Hing himself rejected the medications. Every time he felt better he would stop taking the medications in order to avoid the side effects.

During the course of our involvement with Mr. Hing in the halfway house, I discussed relapse prevention with him. I helped him and his family members (i.e., two sisters) understand his pattern of relapse, and I also discussed how they could better prevent Mr. Hing's relapse and manage the symptoms. Another important discussion was about their views on medication. I acknowledged that the medications had side effects, but I also informed them that without medications Mr. Hing might relapse. Indeed, after some lengthy discussion over a period of time he was able to see the connection between stopping medication and the occurrence of his relapses. However, his sisters insisted on combining Western and alternative medicines, so I provided them with information about the effects and side effects of the medications and invited them to consult Mr. Hing's psychiatrist regarding the intake of Western and alternative medicines. In the first three months of his stay at the halfway house, Mr. Hing appeared to gain mental stability. Although he expressed that he still heard the voice from time to time, he was not distressed by the voice.

Personal Protectors and Risk Factors

Mr. Hing had rather low self-esteem. He held very negative views about himself, particularly regarding his wry neck that he believed was "incurable." The failed efforts to cure his problems, the recurrent relapses, and his failure to be openly employed had confirmed his beliefs about himself (i.e., that he was good-for-nothing). Mr. Hing did not see anything positive about himself and gave up the right to make decisions. This was quite evident when his sisters were around. He would just listen without offering any views or ideas. Mr. Hing had no major skills deficit besides assertiveness.

One of the tasks that the key worker did with Mr. Hing was explore his interests and goals. It became quite obvious that Mr. Hing wanted to find a full-time job as an office worker. He had an eleventh grade education and had learned bookkeeping and typing in the past. The key worker, Mr. Hing, and I discussed the possibility of putting Mr. Hing through office-work training in a day training center. He underwent a work assessment and received training in office work in the following three months. His occupational therapist also encouraged him to learn to be a receptionist and an operator. This turned out to be a possible area of office work for Mr. Hing. He was subsequently given a chance to be placed and later employed at a welfare agency as a part-time operator.

Environmental Stress and Protectors

Throughout the process, workers in the halfway houses were cognizant of any environmental stress that could overwhelm Mr. Hing (i.e., walking on a tightrope). Therefore, Mr. Hing was not pushed to do anything he was not psychologically prepared to do. The workers discussed each step of the rehabilitation process with Mr. Hing and he was given the freedom to do each step at his own pace. Since he took medication regularly (personal protector), his mental state was stabilized. His medications did not need to be adjusted as he took on new initiatives such as working in the day training center and the placement at the welfare agency.

Family climate was a major environmental stress for Mr. Hing. In fact, one reason why he was referred to our halfway house was because of the presence of high expressed emotions in his family. His sisters were overly involved and his mother was very critical of his behavior. In fact, she often nagged him by saying, "Smarten up and get a better job; you should be able to do better than staying in a place for the 'dumb' people." Mr. Hing was able to tell me that he felt distressed by his mother's criticisms and incessant nagging. However, although he felt uncomfortable letting his sisters make every decision for him, he did not say anything. In fact, he did not realize that these actions by his sisters might have seriously undermined his self-esteem.

I conducted a number of family interviews with Mr. Hing's family. His sisters and the mother attended the sessions, but his father never came to any of the interviews. Strategically, we decided to talk about Mr. Hing's mental illness and provided the family with information about the causes and treatment of the illness. We also discussed Mr. Hing's rehabilitation plan, particularly in relation to his plan to find a job as an office worker. This was well received by all members of the family. We gradually moved on to other issues such as the sisters' views of Western and traditional Chinese medications and their enthusiasm in making decisions for Mr. Hing. We commended the sisters and the mother for trying their best to help Mr. Hing, but we also invited Mr. Hing to tell the family his own views. Surprisingly, the sisters were quite willing to let their brother learn to make decisions for himself. As for the mother, she started to understand Mr. Hing's illness and was willing to try not to be too critical of her son. In fact, the two sisters were helpful in teaching their mother to be more accepting. The family members were basically caring and supportive of one another (we knew little about the father, but heard that he was quiet and not very involved in family affairs), and, therefore, the process was enjoyable and positive for all involved.

This chapter has provided a detailed assessment and intervention framework for working with people suffering from schizophrenia. The biological, psychological, and social risk factors and protectors influencing the client's rehabilitation should be examined. When helping a client design and implement a rehabilitation plan it is important to bear in mind the guidelines for working with persons with schizophrenia. A great deal of care must be taken to help the client achieve positive changes while minimizing the amount of stress placed on him or her. Only then can schizophrenia be successfully treated.

Chapter 7

Personality Disorders

INTRODUCTION

Personality is defined as a stable and consistent structure of an individual, characterized by patterns of feelings, thoughts, and behaviors (Kendall & Hammen, 1995). It is shaped by both inborn temperament and social and environmental influences. In fact, a person's personality is expressed in his or her everyday routine interactions. Each individual has a unique personality profile.

When a person's personality profile is considered a disorder, it denotes a persistent pattern of thinking and behaviors that is inflexible, maladaptive, and pervasive across a broad range of personal and social situations. Such patterns lead to significant distress and impairments in a client's functioning (American Psychiatric Association, 2000). Ten types of personality disorders (PDs) exist, which are outlined later in the chapter. Personality disorders are different from one another in terms of their distinctive traits manifested in the clients' thinking, behavior, and feelings. For example, a person with paranoid PD has distinctive character traits such as a distrust of others, and is constantly suspicious of others' motives and argumentativeness. A client with narcissistic PD sees himself or herself as someone who is special and unique and others as inferior. He or she has little regard for rules and is competitive and manipulative.

Personality disorders differ from other forms of psychiatric illnesses because they may not have a strong biophysiological origin (Livesley, 2001). Indeed, no clear biological basis exists for the occurrence of personality disorders. This leads to the question of whether PDs should be seen as problems or as disorders. Controversy exists regarding whether these individuals should be considered as having a mental illness, and about whether people with inflexible behaviors and thinking who are not socially acceptable should be considered as having a medical problem and be treated with medications. Experience shows that only very few cases have biological causes for which medication would be an effective treatment. Many people with PDs have long-standing personality problems that are closely related to lifelong social and environmental influences. Therefore, psychosocial interventions are often more helpful than medicine for modifying their dysfunctional personality traits.

According to the *Hong Kong Rehabilitation Programme Plan Review* (Health and Welfare Bureau, 1999), about 40,000 people suffer from PDs, and of these numbers, 10 percent are receiving psychiatric rehabilitation services. Many people with PDs seek psychiatric services for other mental health problems such as depression, anxiety disorders, or stress-related problems. It usually takes a worker some time before realizing that his or her client's underlying problems are related to personality issues and are not depression or anxiety problems. In other words, the person's depression is primarily a product of his or her personality problems. For example, a woman diagnosed as having depression was referred to me for counseling, and after a few sessions it became apparent that her frequent relationship problems with her boyfriend, colleagues, and mother were related to her dependent personality traits and not to depression. Essentially, she felt she could not survive on her own and that others must always save her. Consequently, she would let others run her life, and became disillusioned when others could not meet all her needs. Gradually, frustrations and despair set in and she became depressed.

Since no direct medical treatment is available for PDs, these individuals are sometimes put on medication for a secondary illness such as depression or an anxiety disorder. In addition, individuals with a PD usually receive counseling from workers and counselors of various social service agencies. Essentially, the major objective of assessment is to understand the client's pattern of behaviors, thinking, and feeling. Counseling should focus on modifying the dysfunctional aspects of the client's personality traits. The word *modifying* is carefully chosen here to denote that personality disorders are difficult to "treat." Oftentimes, the client's personality has developed since childhood and he or she may not see the need to change his or her personality. Moreover, the pattern may become so ingrained that the person must make tremendous efforts to modify his or her behaviors, thinking, and feelings.

ASSESSMENT

Medical Aspects

History of the Client's Personality Traits

It is important to obtain a thorough history of the client's personality development. This helps to distinguish personality disorders (Axis II) from clinical (Axis I) mental disorders, based on the DSM-IV-TR. A person diagnosed as having a PD must exhibit personality traits that have developed since childhood, and that are typical of his or her long-term functioning. Second, and more important, this history-taking exercise can help the worker identify the client's pattern of thinking, behaviors, and feelings. Particularly, it is useful to understand how and why these patterns are being sustained. This information helps the worker help the client (1) understand his or her pattern of thinking, behaving, and feeling, and how this pattern affects his functioning; and (2) find the maintenance factors that perpetuate the pattern.

Understanding maladaptive patterns. A client with PD normally does not have much insight into his or her personality problems. These traits have been a part of his or her makeup since childhood. Unless the client genuinely gains insight into his or her personality problems, he or she is not likely to attempt to make any change. For example, after seeing me for a few months, one of my clients with antisocial personality disorder began to talk about his fear of losing the right to visit his son, who was in the custody of his ex-wife. He realized his angry outbursts could jeopardize his allowed access, and he also felt that his misbehaviors could become a bad model for his child. Consequently, he was more willing to work to find ways of managing his anger and frustration.

Finding patterns of behavior. Despite that many personality problems bring forth psychosocial difficulties for clients, many continue to hold on to their patterns. Two possible reasons can be given for this. First, a client gains benefits from engaging in such behaviors, thoughts, and feelings. Second, the client's pattern has become so habitual that he or she automatically relates and responds to others in their negative fashion. For example, a client of mine with borderline personality disorder wanted to keep her husband from divorcing her, and she avoided abandonment by attempting to overdose. When I saw her, she had already attempted suicide more than ten times. Her strong fear of abandonment and her insecurity had driven her to make all efforts to control her relationships with men (she had had several relationships). However, she did this by blackmailing her boyfriends and by attempting suicide. Through these acts, my client thought she could sense her boyfriends' worries and get some "reassurance" from them. Even though these tactics failed eventually, such behaviors were reinforced by the immediate sense of relief and false security. Moreover, she had become accustomed to behaving in such a way, and thus, whenever she experienced a sense of abandonment, she automatically resorted to committing suicide as a way of keeping her boyfriends.

Coexistence of Psychiatric Illness

As mentioned previously, a client with PD may exhibit other psychiatric symptoms such as depressed moods, anxiety, and delusions. It is necessary to distinguish whether the client has an Axis I disorder, such as depression or anxiety disorder, because it is possible that the person with an Axis I diagnosis has an underlying personality problem. Indeed, such an Axis I disorder may originate from or be closely related to an Axis II personality disorder (American Psychiatric Association, 2000). For example, I have had clients who came to see me for an Axis I disorder (e.g., depression), but turned out to have underlying personality problems needing much attention. In these circumstances, it is not possible to address the Axis I disorder without first focusing on the long-standing personality problems. For example, a man who had been diagnosed with depression was referred to me for counseling, and it soon became apparent that he too often questioned the intentions of others and accused others of playing tricks on him. He felt very distressed at work and complained that his boss and colleagues were trying to kick him out of his job. Consequently, he became depressed. In my opinion, the client's depression (Axis I) was very much linked to his paranoid personality traits (Axis II). He was given medication by the psychiatrist, and he was also provided with counseling to understand and modify his paranoid personality traits.

Medications

It is important to state here that no medication exists that can treat PDs. However, some people with PDs are put on medication. In these circumstances, medications are often prescribed to relieve symptoms of other psychiatric illnesses, such as depression and anxiety disorders. It is therefore useful for the worker to know what types of medication the client is taking. Moreover, the worker must ensure that the client clearly understands why he or she is taking the medication as well as the effects and side effects of the medication.

Profile of Personality Disorders

DSM-IV-TR (American Psychiatric Association, 2000) classifies personality disorders according to the distinctive behavioral manifestations of each type of disorder. Broadly speaking, these behavioral manifestations can be classified into three categories: odd-eccentric, dramatic-emotional, and anxious-fearful. Paranoid, schizoid, and schizotypal PD are grouped under Cluster A (odd-eccentric); antisocial, borderline, histrionic, and narcissistic PD are put under Cluster B (dramatic-emotional); and avoidant, dependent, and obsessive-compulsive PD are grouped in Cluster C (anxious-fearful).

Cluster A

Paranoid personality disorder. Clients with paranoid PD are distrustful and suspicious of others, persistently bear grudges, are reluctant to confide in others, and have recurrent suspicions, without justification, regarding the fidelity of spouse or sexual partner. For example, a client of mine diagnosed as having paranoid PD was generally and persistently distrustful of others, made many complaints about different people, and was very suspicious of the fidelity of his wife. He followed her everywhere, and on a few occasions even hit her, thinking that she was having an affair with another man.

Schizoid personality disorder. People with this type of PD have a persistent pattern of detachment from social relationships and a restricted range of emotional expression. Indeed, these clients are loners, indifferent to approval or criticism, and do not appear to be bothered by what others think of them. For example, one thirty-one-year-old man with schizoid PD who had lived on his own before being referred by the hospital to our halfway house did not talk to anyone and refused to participate in any social activities. Moreover, he did not enjoy mixing with others and appeared rather self-sufficient. He wore very thick clothes even in the hot summer days. In the halfway house, he was given the nickname "Hermit the frog" by other residents.

Schizotypal personality disorder. These individuals have marked deficits in social and interpersonal relationships. They feel particularly uncomfortable and anxious in social situations and exhibit eccentric behaviors. They lack close friends and confidants, and may also have odd beliefs or magical thinking. Unlike people with schizoid PD who do not enjoy and refuse to enter relationships, people with schizotypal PD still participate in social relationships even though they experience much anxiety and discomfort.

Cluster B

Antisocial personality disorder. People with antisocial PD have pervasive patterns of disregard for and violation of the rights of others, occurring since the age of fifteen. They normally exhibit conduct problems during childhood. These individuals may be deceitful, impulsive, irritable, and aggressive. Moreover, they do not show any remorse for their misbehaviors. For example, one of my clients, a typical person with antisocial PD, had since childhood been in and out of the legal system and had repeatedly broken the law. He was impulsive and became irritable very easily. He would also act aggressively when he felt he was provoked. On one occasion, when one of our staff did not let him do something he wanted to do, he became so angry that he not only raised his voice but threw a chair at this particular staff member. He later admitted to much more drastic and aggressive behavior in the past when he lost his temper.

Borderline personality disorder. People with this disorder often engage in unstable and intense interpersonal relationships. They have a strong fear of abandonment, an unstable self-image, and are impulsive. These individuals are emotionally unstable with marked changes in mood. They have recurrent suicidal ideas, suicidal attempts, and inflict deliberate self-harm. One client having a typical case of borderline personality disorder often came to my office with excessive and intense emotions. She was first referred to me after her eleventh suicide attempt. As she expressed, "I was very unhappy and I could not bear the worries and unhappiness of having the thought of him leaving me. I had no choice but to end my life."

Histrionic personality disorder. These individuals want to be the center of attention, and engage in inappropriate sexually seductive or provocative behaviors. They also use physical appearance to draw others' attention and display self-dramatization and exaggerated expression of emotions. I had a client who was referred to me after an overdose. A home visit revealed that her whole apartment was full of Marilyn Monroe memorabilia. Indeed, she dressed glamorously and appeared rather seductive in an attempt to be similar to her idol. Her physical appearance and speech were excessively impressionistic and "shallow."

Narcissistic personality disorder. Those with narcissistic PD have a grandiose sense of self-importance and are preoccupied with fantasies of unlimited power, success, and achievement. They lack empathy and are exploitative in relationships. Indeed, they appear very arrogant to others.

Cluster C

Avoidant personality disorder. People with this PD feel inadequate, are hypersensitive to negative criticism, and are unwilling to get involved with people unless they feel well-liked. They are reluctant to take personal risks or to engage in any new adventures because of the fear of embarrassment.

Dependent personality disorder. These individuals have excessive need to be protected by others, exhibit submissive and clingy behavior, and are afraid of separation. They have difficulty making everyday decisions and asserting themselves. They seek another relationship as a source of care when a close relationship ends. A thirty-year-old client of mine had just broken up with her boyfriend and became rather depressed. This was her third time experiencing depression as a result of a separation. She said she felt very lonely and did not have someone to "rely on." She could not bear to make decisions for herself. She also blamed herself for all the breakups and said, "They told me that I should be more independent and give them room to breathe. But I have been like this all my life."

Obsessive-compulsive personality disorder. Individuals with this PD have a preoccupation with orderliness, perfection, and a sense of control. They look for details, rules, and schedules, and are overly conscientious and inflexible about matters of morality and ethics. They are rigid and stubborn.

Medical Interventions

Not a great deal of medical options are available for treating people with PDs, and no medication exists that can treat PDs per se. However, medications are often prescribed to treat Axis I diseases that accompany PDs. For example, PD clients may be prescribed antidepressants and antianxiety medications. Therefore, the worker needs to educate the client about the effects and side effects of these medications. Moreover, since such clients may not need continuous medications, the worker should monitor their medications carefully by negotiating with the psychiatrists regarding any change in a client's circumstances.

Cognitive and Behavioral Aspects

Beck et al. (1990) provide a cognitive-behavioral framework for understanding and working with people with PDs. Several assumptions can be made when working with PDs, which are outlined in the following section.

Basic Assumptions

Dysfunctional feelings and conduct are due to certain cognitive schemas that tend to produce consistently biased judgments and persistent misbehaviors (Beck et al., 1990). For example, since a person with paranoid PD views others as malicious and having ill intentions, he or she will judge and react to people's behaviors in a biased manner.

Patterned thinking and behaviors are learned throughout childhood. It is therefore necessary to get a detailed history of the person's patterns of thinking and behavior. Particularly, the worker must help the client understand how his or her perceptions have created biased judgments toward others, how his or her judgments influence his or her behavior, and how the responses from others have reinforced such perceptions. For instance, a person with schizoid PD has formed the opinion that interpersonal relationships are unrewarding and therefore he or she does not initiate and maintain relationships with others. Lacking the adequate skills and motivations to mix with others, he or she does not receive positive interpersonal responses from others. Consequently, his or her negative views about interpersonal relationships are reinforced. It is necessary to help the client find ways to break this vicious cycle.

Different types of personality disorders have distinctive thought, emotional, and behavioral patterns. These can be categorized under core beliefs, dysfunctional rules, and maladaptive coping behaviors. Indeed, it is even more appropriate to say that each individual has his or her unique set of thinking and behaviors and that the worker should examine each person individually.

The focus of change centers around core personality problems (schematic) and not on symptoms (Beck et al., 1990). Generally speaking, cognitive approaches are quite effective in symptom management of people with depression and anxiety disorders. However, in the case of people with PDs, the central intervention focus shifts to modifying the core beliefs of the individuals. Symptom management is deemphasized.

PD clients are unaware of their problems. Many do not realize that they have a maladaptive pattern of thinking and behaving. Nor can they see the link between their patterns and their personal difficulties. Psychoeducation is an important strategy in arousing the clients' awareness of their problems.

Patterned thinking and behaviors are more resistant to change. It has taken clients with PDs years to develop their patterns of thinking and behaviors. They also receive secondary gains in the process. Therefore, it will take a long time for people with PDs to unlearn their patterns and acquire more adaptive patterns of thinking and behaviors. The worker needs to use different strategies to help the clients understand how their thoughts and behaviors affect their lives and to modify their maladaptive thoughts and behaviors.

Assessment

In the assessment, the worker needs to identify a client's pattern of (1) core beliefs (2) dysfunctional rules, and (3) maladaptive coping strategies. Based on the work of Beck et al. (1990), cognitive profiles of each type of PD are outlined in the following paragraphs.

Paranoid PD. People with this type of PD think that they are righteous and that they are vulnerable to being cheated by others. They view others as malicious and having abusive motives. As a result, they have developed the rules of "Never trust anyone," "Be on guard or else be cheated," and "Every person's action has a malicious motive." In order to protect themselves, these individuals develop negative behavioral responses such as constantly looking for hidden motives, accusing others of malice, and being extremely cautious.

Schizoid PD. These individuals perceive themselves as self-sufficient and without need of others. They consider any attempt by others to involve them as intrusive. They have dysfunctional rules such as "Relationships are unrewarding" and "My life is better without others." Essentially, they resort to staying away from others as much as possible.

Schizotypal PD. People with this type of PD function under such beliefs as "I am different" and "No one understands me." They have dysfunctional rules such as "Since no one understands me, I just do what I think is right" and "I never fit into the social norms." As far as maladaptive coping skills are concerned, these individuals continue to engage in the eccentric behaviors they think are right and avoid entering interpersonal relationships in which they feel uncomfortable.

Antisocial PD. Clients with antisocial PD see themselves as extremely strong and cannot tolerate the thought of anyone hindering them from getting exactly what they want. Therefore, those who are perceived as stopping them from fulfilling their needs deserve to be punished. They have developed dysfunctional rules such as "I am not responsible for any wrongdoing" and "I must act before others attack me." As far as maladaptive coping strategies are concerned, they try to engage in attacking, deceiving, and manipulating others.

Borderline PD. These individuals see themselves as empty and void. They also hold a strong belief that people close to them will eventually desert them. Under the influence of these beliefs, they develop dysfunctional rules such as "If I do not cling to my loved ones they will abandon me," and "If people refuse to do as I say, they do not love me or care about me." Behaviorally, these individuals use all the methods they can think of to make sure that their loved ones will not abandon them, including suicide attempts. They will also try to manipulate others by expressing intense emotions toward them.

Histrionic PD. Those with histrionic PD have a strong belief that they are the center of attention, and deserve this attention because they are glamorous and impressive. Others should admire them and can be seduced by them. They have such dysfunctional rules as "People are here to serve me and admire me" and "No one should undermine me." These individuals may act dramatically, using charm, temper tantrums, and suicidal gestures to get what they want.

Narcissistic PD. These individuals believe that they are special, unique, and superior. On the same note, they believe others are inferior and should be treated accordingly. They hold such dysfunctional rules as "since I am special, I deserve special rules" and "I am better than others." As far as maladaptive coping strategies are concerned, these people are manipulative and competitive. They use others and disregard them at the same time.

Avoidant PD. People with avoidant PD see themselves as socially inept and are vulnerable to criticism and rejection. They see others as critical, demeaning, and superior. The have developed such rules as "I must avoid others because they will put me down." and "If people know the real me, they will reject me." Understandably, these individuals engage in avoidance behaviors and do not enter into social contact or interpersonal relationships.

Dependent PD. These clients believe that they are weak and incompetent, and that they are helpless without others. On the other hand, others are nurturing, supportive, and competent. They hold such dysfunctional rules as "I cannot survive without others" and "I need to be constantly nurtured or I cannot go on." These individuals seek advice all the times, do not make decisions for themselves, and let others run their lives. Moreover, they are unassertive and yield to authority or request very easily.

Obsessive-compulsive PD. These people see themselves as responsible, competent, and fastidious. They perceive others as irresponsible, incompetent, and casual. These individuals have many rigid and dysfunctional rules, such as "It is important to know every detail. Otherwise, things will not work out" and "People should work harder and be more serious." In terms of maladaptive coping strategies, these individuals constantly evaluate and criticize others. They engage in constant "should" thinking and behaviors. Last, they adhere rather rigidly to rules and do not tolerate ambiguity.

INTERVENTIONS

Relationship Building

A close and warm relationship between client and worker is necessary for intervention (Turkat, 1990). This is the most important part of the intervention process; however, it is not easy to engage people with PD in the therapeutic process. Often these individuals manifest a variety of testing behaviors to find out how much the worker cares about him or her and to find the worker's limits. A directive stance is often successful, done by verbally expressing concerns for the clients and providing them with instrumental assistance. However, if and when clients' behaviors exceed the worker's level of tolerance, he or she can point out the client's misbehaviors and explain how and why the behaviors cannot be accepted. The client should be told how others might perceive and respond to those behaviors as well. For example, a twenty-five-year-old young man with a rather disruptive childhood was referred to our halfway house. He acted out by pounding on the tables and making loud noises whenever he felt frustrated and unhappy. Although I tried to empathize with his unhappiness and grief over the fear of abandonment, I told him that his behavior greatly disturbed me and others in the house. I told him that I cared about him but could not tolerate such misbehavior. It is important for the worker to understand that he or she needs to show concern for the clients but must also be firm and assertive.

Noncollaboration is very common (Turkat, 1990). The worker must be prepared for clients with PD who are resistant to change and, in fact, may consciously or unconsciously try to sabotage the change. Noncollaboration occurs for a few reasons. First, clients do not see the need to change. Since their patterned ways of thinking and behaviors have survival value, they need to see and feel that there are strong and pervasive reasons for them to change. For example, a person with dependent PD engages in his or her way of thinking and behaving in order to feel that he or she is being taken care of by others. Throughout the process, the person actually receives emotional and instrumental support from others. Unless strong and overriding reasons for change are discovered, it is not easy for him or her to have the courage to change his or her personality pattern. Second, these patterns of thinking and behaving have become automatic responses. It would take a great deal of effort for them to consciously be aware of these responses and to stop them at appropriate moments.

Transference and countertransference are evident among people with PDs (Walsh, 2000). *Transference* happens when the client relates to the worker in the same problematic ways as he or she relates to others. For example, a person with dependent PD makes the worker an object of dependence and allows the worker to make decisions for him or her. Countertransference occurs when the worker becomes angry and frustrated with the client, and loses his or her composure. For example, a worker working with a person with dependent PD may become frustrated because the client keeps asking the worker to make decisions for him or her despite constant reminders that the client must make his or her own decisions. The worker needs to be aware of the possibility of any transference or countertransference, and must work through his or her own feelings. Since the worker handling clients with PDs often experiences countertransference, he or she should learn ways of handling their own emotions. One way is to talk to and seek advice from colleagues and/or superviors when he or she feels frustrated with clients.

Limit setting is necessary. Some people with dependent, histrionic, antisocial, and borderline PDs may engage in behaviors that test the limits of the worker. Although the worker must have concern for the individuals, he or she needs to set limits on their behaviors, otherwise they will become more and more difficult to handle. The important goal to bear in mind is consistency. The worker should uphold the limits as much as possible, and should be cognizant of the different ways that clients test the limits.

Facilitating Client's Awareness of PD

As mentioned before, many clients with PDs are not aware of the severity of their problems, and due to secondary gains they continue to think, feel, and behave in certain maladaptive ways. The first step in counseling those with PDs is to help them understand and feel motivated to make certain changes.

Conceptualizing and Educating the Client

Through the initial interviews, the worker needs to find the connections between core beliefs, dysfunctional rules, and maladaptive coping strategies. The worker must also identify the vicious cycle and maintenance factors associated with the person's PD and should educate the client about these connections. It is useful to employ a conceptualization diagram to help the client understand these various issues (see Figure 5.2 in Chapter 5). No fixed way of constructing a conceptualization diagram exists; the worker needs to identify the connections and draw out the flow systematically while discussing it with the client.

Understanding the Client's Underlying Yearnings

A client with PD must see a need for change. Generally speaking, it is assumed that people interact and respond to the external environment in ways that would help them fulfill their needs. In Glasser's (1984) classification, these needs include the need to belong, the need for power, the need for freedom, and the need for fun. An important task for the worker is to unearth a client's underlying yearnings that are connected to his or her present maladaptive behaviors, thinking, and emotions. The worker should also explain that the client's present response pattern will not and cannot help fulfill his or her underlying yearnings. In essence, one way of helping clients identify a reason for change is to help them realize that their old patterns of response will not get them what they want in life.

In the case of the aforementioned client with antisocial PD, he yearned for the love of others but became frustrated easily when people did not fulfill his needs immediately. Since his wife did not approve of his full access right to his son, he showed a great deal of anger aggression toward her. I pointed out that although his thought of maintaining access to his son was amicable (i.e., an act of love), his behaviors toward his wife would not help him fulfill his needs. Since seeing his son was something that he really wanted, he was willing to work with me in modifying his temper.

Modifying the Client's Pattern of Responses

Guided Discovery

The worker can use the daily dysfunctional thoughts worksheet (see Figure 4.2 in Chapter 4), diaries, or guided imagery to help the client come to an understanding of his or her pattern of maladaptive thinking and behaviors (Beck, 1995). The worker should instruct the client to record the necessary information on the worksheet or in a diary, or should ask the client to recall certain incidents in his or her mind to guide the client in making connections between feelings, thinking, and behaviors. The worker should show the client how these various responses have contributed to his or her emotional problems. Ideally, the client will self-discover and the worker will simply assist him or her in arriving at his or her own conclusion. Thus, the worker should avoid directly pointing out the connection for the client, but should instead raise questions throughout the process. Otherwise, the client may feel that the worker forcibly put thoughts into his or her mind.

Creating Opportunities

Another direction of guided discovery is to create opportunities for a client to self-examine his or her thoughts, behaviors, and emotions, and to experiment with new ways of thinking and behaving. For example, a female client with dependent PD was asked to take note of her behaviors, thoughts, and emotions toward her husband (her husband had become rather frustrated with her) and of the resultant responses of her husband. We examined the various events thoroughly and discussed how she might respond differently. She was also requested to note her husband's subsequent set of responses. It is important to bear in mind that a client with PD needs many opportunities to examine and test new patterns of responses. The worker and the client must work hard to identify and structure these opportunities. No one can talk another person out of his or her beliefs, and any change in perception must be accompanied by new experiences that contravene the person's long-held beliefs.

Working Through Client's Transference

A client may engage in transference and display his or her pattern of thinking, behavior, and feeling onto the worker. The worker can use the process of transference to point out the client's maladaptive pattern of responses and can discuss the various feelings he or she has toward the client's transference. This real and experiential exercise can be very revealing to the client. For example, a client with antisocial PD on one occasion was verbally aggressive toward me. Fortunately, I managed to calm him down. At the end of that interview, I disclosed how fearful and uncomfortable the verbal abuse made me and how others in the same situation might have felt about him.

Confronting the Client's Schemas and Misbehaviors

Sometimes, the worker may want to directly confront the client about his or her maladaptive responses (Beck et al., 1990). Both the client and the worker may not feel comfortable with this direct confrontation; however, when this is done in a concerned manner, the client may in fact appreciate the openness of the worker. Although the client may not immediately accept the worker's confrontation, he or she can tell when the worker is genuinely concerned about him or her and appreciates the worker's constructive criticism.

GUIDELINES FOR WORKING WITH PERSONS WITH PERSONALITY DISORDERS

The focus of intervention centers on modifying a client's pattern of cognition, behavior, and emotion.

Because the pattern has been developed since childhood or adolescence, it takes a great deal of time and many opportunities for the client to successfully modify his or her pattern of responses. The ultimate goal of counseling is to help the client modify his or her patterns of thinking, behavior, and feeling so that his or her responses can be less disturbing to oneself and others.

A good worker-client relationship is essential for successful intervention.

This is not an understatement. It is important for the client to feel that the worker is genuinely concerned about him or her. Otherwise, confrontation may become counterproductive. Without a good relationship, the client may not even try to make the change and comply with the limits set by the worker.

The worker should anticipate problems with compliance.

People with PDs do not want to or cannot easily change their patterns of thinking and behavior. They may consciously or unconsciously sabotage the worker's and their own efforts. The worker needs to be patient with the client and deal with the issue of countertransference.

A client may engage in transference and display various emotions.

It is necessary for the worker to be aware of and to find ways of helping the client understand how transference may be affecting their relationships and how the client's usual response pattern may be detrimental to oneself and others.

Limit setting is important.

People with PDs may test the limits of their behaviors. A worker needs to be aware of the various intents of the client in crossing the limits, and respond by setting certain limits to the person's behaviors. This is an important negotiation process that the client needs to learn so that he or she does not resort to an automatic but often drastic and destructive response pattern.

CASE ILLUSTRATION

Nigel was a thirty-seven-year-old man who worked as an electrician. He was single and was clinically depressed with symptoms of sleeplessness, poor appetite, and low moods. He was diagnosed as having depression and referred to me for counseling, particularly on issues related to his house and the relationship with his girlfriend. However, it soon caught my attention that Nigel appeared to have a repeated pattern of how he perceived and related to others and that he was very unhappy with those experiences. Indeed, I consulted the psychiatrist on our team and we felt that Nigel had very persistent personality traits that fell into the paranoid PD category.

I invited Nigel to tell me about his past. He said he had lived alone for years. His parents were still alive. He described his father as an "invalid" who had a long-standing depression and portrayed his mother as very detached and domineering. He mentioned that he had a very isolated childhood and had never developed any close relationships with others. Indeed, he did not feel safe with others and felt that no one would protect and help him.

Medical Aspect

Nigel was put on antidepressant, dothiepin, 75 mg daily. He claimed that he did not feel a difference after taking the medication. Indeed, he wanted to stop the medication as soon as possible. Nigel had just moved into the new neighborhood and joined his girlfriend, who had brought a house next to him. The first few counseling sessions became his platform for complaining about other people. He complained about the city council, saying that council staff were pushing him. He also blamed the previous owner for selling him such a shabby house that required immediate repair works. He held grudges against his girlfriend for encouraging him to move into the area, and he was angry with his supervisor for being very bossy and controlling. Underneath these complaints, Nigel felt that people were malicious and intended to take advantage of him. Indeed, he felt that he was an innocent victim for many things that happened in his life. Since he had so much anger and frustration, I intended to give him as much room to air out his unhappiness as possible. Moreover, I did not question the validity of his complaints, but empathized with his unhappiness. It seemed that he was quite comfortable with me and was willing to tell me his thoughts and feelings. However, in the beginning of the counseling sessions, it became apparent that Nigel would disagree with anything I, and perhaps anyone, suggested. I decided that I would not offer him any advice or suggestions, but instead encourage him to give the answers himself. This strategy turned out to be useful in handling people such as Nigel. He did not see me as having any hidden motive nor did he feel that I had any intention of getting anything from him or of siding with anyone to take advantage of him.

Cognitive and Behavioral Aspects

Nigel had core beliefs that he was innocent and vulnerable, and that others were malicious and would take advantage of him. He interpreted others' actions as having hidden motives. His dysfunctional rules were quite obvious, being "Do not trust anyone" and "Be always on guard." As far as his maladaptive coping strategies were concerned, he always looked for hidden motives and accused people of trying to take advantage of him.

The most difficult part of the intervention was helping Nigel examine how his pattern of thinking and behavior might have direct bearing on his distress. When Nigel spoke of the events of his childhood and adolescence, I often asked him, "How did this affect you?" He was able to realize that he did not trust people, but was adamant that people were largely unworthy of being trusted. I then invited him to consider whether his lack of trust in others had anything to do with his unhappiness and whether it was worth holding on to such character traits. However, I did acknowledge that his experiences were real to him, and that unless he had other experiences that could counteract these, he would continue to distrust others.

One of the major sources of his complaints was related to his relationship with his supervisor. He felt that his supervisor was trying to trick him so that he might loss his job. Since Nigel was eager to keep his job, he was willing to discuss the matter with me and participated in the process. I invited him to write down the evidence that supported his claim. When he produced the materials in the later counseling sessions, we discussed the evidence. In the process, I did not deny his perceptions of the evidence. On the other hand, I often asked him to suggest possible (though to him unreal) alternative interpretations of the evidence he had. As time passed, Nigel felt a bit more relaxed with his supervisor. Since he had recovered from his depression and did not need to take the medication, he decided to stop counseling as well. I did not think that he had changed his paranoid personality traits, but he certainly had gained some understanding of how his paranoid personality traits had affected his ways of thinking and behaviors. Moreover, he was less rigid than before.

This chapter has delineated an assessment and intervention framework for working with people suffering from personality disorders. Different types of personality disorders have distinctive thought, emotional, and behavioral patterns that can be categorized under negative core beliefs, dysfunctional rules, and maladaptive coping behaviors. A worker needs to help the client identify these patterns and develop strategies to alter his or her thoughts and behaviors. It is essential to remember the following points when working with a client with PD: build a good relationship, accept noncollaboration, be aware of transference and countertransference, and set limits with the client.

Chapter 8

Working with Families

INTRODUCTION

The number of individuals suffering from mental illness who are living with family members in Hong Kong is unknown. In China, Phillips, Xiong, & Zhao (1990) estimate that more than 90 percent of such individuals live with their family members. This is a realistic estimation because of the scarcity of community residential facilities for people with mental illness in China. In the United States, Hatfield and Lefley (1987) suggest that the number is about 20 to 65 percent. Since young adults in the United States tend to leave home early and live independently, Hatfield and Lefley's estimation is credible. In present-day Hong Kong it can be estimated that the number of individuals with chronic mental illness who are living with families is about 80 to 90 percent. This rough calculation is based on subtracting the number of persons with severe mental illness living in different residential facilities from the total estimated population of individuals with severe mental illness as stated in the *Hong Kong Rehabilitation Programme Plan Review* (Health and Welfare Bureau, 1999). This figure deserves attention because many studies have revealed that family members who live and care for relatives suffering from serious mental illness experience a high level of stress and poor mental health (Noh & Turner, 1987; Wong, 2000). Such family members often do not have the necessary caring and management skills to handle relatives with mental illness. This is particularly relevant for families in Hong Kong because of the lack of social services for caregivers. Very few government-subsidized family resource centers and self-funded family organizations are available for family members in Hong Kong. Indeed, many family caregivers do not receive any services from the community in Hong Kong (Wong, Pui, Pearson, & Chiu, 2003).

UNDERSTANDING THE ROLES AND REACTIONS OF FAMILY MEMBERS

Current Views

In the past thirty years, a shift has occurred in perceptions and attitudes about the role of family members regarding the causation of mental illness found in their relatives with serious mental illness. *Schizophrenogenic mothers* is a term used to describe the theory that cold and controlling mothers alienated their children and caused them to suffer from schizophrenia. *Double-bind hypothesis* suggests that conflicting and inconsistent expectations within the family that a child cannot meet will cause him or her to develop schizophrenia. *Marital schism* refers to children who grew up in families with a high level of marital conflicts, causing a child to have split loyalties and thus develop schizophrenia (Hatfield & Lefley, 1987). However, none of the previous three theories received adequate empirical support when they were proposed and thus were not favored by academic communities. On the other hand, empirical evidence suggests that family members suffer from physical and mental health problems as a result of rendering care continuously to their relatives with mental illness. The notion that family members cause mental illness has come under challenge and has been reformulated to include a more balanced view of families instead being resources and partners in the caring process. As a consequence, attention given to understanding and establishing direct services for family members with relatives suffering from serious mental illness has increased. To conclude, the perceptions toward family members have shifted from that of a contributor to that of a sufferer (i.e., they did not not cause the illness but are also suffering because of the illness), from a person with problems to a person with resources, and from a recipient of service to a partner in care.

Stages of Psychological Reactions and Implications for Interventions

Literature suggests that family members, particularly the primary caregivers, go through different stages of psychological reactions to having a relative suffering from serious mental illness. These include denial, guilt and self-blame, overreliance on mental health professionals, realization of the chronicity of the illness, and constant fear and anxiety about their relatives future (Torrey, 1988; Bernheim & Lehman, 1985; Hatfield & Lefley, 1987). However, it must be stressed that family caregivers do not necessarily go through all the stages of psychological reactions outlined in the following sections. Nor do all families with relatives suffering from mental illness have to go through these psychological reactions. Nonetheless, this stage perspective provides a general framework and possible focuses for intervention to help mental health workers understand the psychological reactions and needs of caregivers.

Denial

Family members may not be fully aware of the signs and symptoms of a mental illness, particularly in the initial phase of its development. It is not uncommon for family members to label the illness in terms of something other than a mental illness. Indeed, many symptoms of a mental illness may initially be interpreted as conduct problems, personality inadequacies, and as reactions to psychosocial stress. Family members of different traditions and cultural origins may also label these signs and symptoms using culturally acquired causes such as possession by evil spirits and imbalance of yin and yang. In my own studies, results repeatedly suggest that many Chinese family members in Hong Kong no longer use traditional cultural labels to interpret the symptoms of a mental illness; they have come to believe that mental illness is caused by the exposure to excessive stress and by personality inadequacies (Wong & Poon, 2002; Wong et al., 2003). Coupled with the heavy stigma placed on mental illness in many cultures, including Hong Kong, family members who are not accustomed to a medical orientation of mental illness may deny the presence of mental illness in their family members. Indeed, the longer the family members deny the presence of mental illness, the greater the family members and relatives with the illness will suffer. During the period of denial, family members struggle to make sense of and cope with the behaviors and emotions of the mentally ill relative. However, without proper treatment, the relative must bear the unpleasant and fear-inducing symptoms. It is important for the worker to tap into their perceptions of mental illness early as possible so that family members can acquire a proper understanding of the causation of mental illness.

Guilt and Self-Blame

It is quite common for family members, particularly parents, to question whether they are somehow responsible for "causing" mental illness in their relatives. Improper childbearing and rearing practices, marital discord, improper diet, and personal misconduct are some of the common reasons for illness that parents suggest in the initial stage of their relatives' mental illness. This sense of guilt can have detrimental effects on the psychological well-being of family members as well as on the rehabilitation of the relative with mental illness. Some family members bearing the psychological burden of having "caused" mental illness tend to overcompensate for their "wrongdoings" by being overprotective of the relative and preventing him or her from engaging in proper rehabilitation services and programs. Therefore, it is important for the worker to explore whether family members, particularly parents, have such feelings of guilt and self-blame. Indeed, a tendency among many families to overprotect their relatives. For example, one client with an adult son with chronic schizophrenia felt that the disease was caused by her poor child-rearing practices and she therefore had to compensate by doing as much as she could to make her son feel better. She would disagree to cooperate with the worker any time her son disliked the worker's suggestion. It became rather difficult for the worker to engage her son in meaningful rehabilitation activities because of the mother's attitude.

Overreliance on Mental Health Professionals

Literature suggests that it takes about a year before family members can identify the correct professionals or psychiatric services to help a relative with mental illness (Chiu, Poon, Fong, & Tsoh, 2000). Many families first rely on close family members for advice, information, and practical assistance. It is only when a relative's illness becomes unmanageable that such families seek help from formal psychiatric services. A lack of understanding of mental illness, a lack of access to psychiatric services, psychiatric stigma, and enclosed family networks are among the major reasons for a delay in help-seeking. However, once family members approach mental health medical professionals for help, they may develop a dependency on the professionals and rely heavily on them for treating their relative's illness. Indeed, family members hope that the mental health professional can cure their relative's illness. This undue faith in the professional may have negative impact on the family members because it may cause them to not be active in caring for their relative. Moreover, they may not develop competence to handle their relative's problems and feel frustrated and disappointed when they realize that their relative's conditions cannot be cured.

Realization of the Chronicity of the Illness

Reality finally strikes family members when a relative with mental illness experiences ongoing residual symptoms, recurrent psychiatric relapses, and/or exhibits disturbing behaviors repeatedly over time. Family members then realize that no cure exists for the many types of serious mental illness and their relative's conditions may possibly deteriorate further in spite of the intake of medications. Moreover, in some cases, family members begin to realize that their relatives can never perform socially and vocationally as well as they once did and that they have become a different person. It takes a few years before family members come to accept the chronicity of a serious mental illness. Whereas some family members are able to accept and perceive this chronicity in a positive light, others react negatively and experience stress and strain in their daily encounters with the relative due to unmet expectations. Mental health workers need to identify these family members and help them work through their lack of recognition and acceptance of the chronicity of mental illness.

Constant Fear of and Anxiety About the Future

One of the stressors that has often been identified in studies on caregivers with relatives suffering from mental illness is the constant fear and anxiety about the future of their relatives (Wong et al., 2003). It is not uncommon to find that family members, particularly parents of older age, mention that they are constantly afraid of the future prospects of their relatives. Their fear is not totally ungrounded because in Hong Kong the waiting list for different types of residential facilities for people with chronic mental illness is very long, and therefore the relative may not have anywhere to stay or someone to provide care when older family members pass away. Mental health workers need to help these family members plan ahead so that the relative with the illness has adequate future arrangements. Moreover, the workers need to help some older family members learn to let go and give their relative a chance to acquire skills for independent living. Nonetheless, the workers must show understanding of the difficulties borne by some family members in relinquishing their involvement. These families may have been so involved that they have not yet understood the importance of training their relative with mental illness to live independently.

Skills for Handling the Psychological Reactions of Family Members

To begin with, it is important for mental health workers to accept and appreciate the difficulties faced by family members. These families need to be reassured that they are doing their best to take care of their relative with the illness as far as their resources, readiness, and willingness are concerned. The worker must start from whatever stage of the process the family members are in and help them to gradually participate as much as they can and are willing to participate. It is necessary for the worker to withhold his or her judgment regarding family members' attitudes and behaviors toward their relative. Instead, the worker needs to see these families as potential resources in rendering care. The skills outlined in the following sections are useful for working with family members.

Listening and Supporting

Family members are human beings too. Some may express intense frustration, anger, and unhappiness during the course of their relative's care. They need someone who is willing to listen to their grievances and who will show them that their concerns are understood. Many times, these families want someone willing to listen rather than someone to give advice. Indeed, once these families feel that they are being understood, they may have the strengths to work on the issues themselves.

Validating

Families need to know that their efforts in caring for their relatives with mental illness are appreciated and helpful. Although family members do not always offer the right type of care and some may in fact be unhelpful to the relatives with mental illness, family members must have done something right if they themselves have sought help. It is important for the workers to identify and validate the appropriate efforts and to encourage family members to do more of them. Encouragement breeds actions that lead to positive changes.

Gentle Guiding

Some family members may be indifferent to the care of their relatives with mental illness. It is important to start at their current level of involvement and gently encourage them to be as involved as they can be. In any case, the workers should not push the families to assume responsibilities that they are not ready or unwilling to assume. In fact, workers must learn to accept that some family members will never be much involved in the caring process.

Clarifying Misunderstanding

Some family members are unwilling to be involved because they have developed negative views of their relative with mental illness. For example, some family members misperceive their relative's negative symptoms as signs of personality inadequacies and claim that the relative should be responsible for his or her problems. Others cannot tolerate the bizarre behaviors and labile moods of their relatives, arguing that they should learn to control these behaviors and emotions. These examples show that family members often do not have adequate understanding of a serious mental illness, such as schizophrenia, and cannot accept them. A worker should take note of this misunderstanding and help family members acquire sufficient knowledge about mental illness.

Helping Family Members Make Realistic Expectations

As previously mentioned, some relatives' mental illnesses may be so disabling that they cannot achieve much improvement in their rehabilitation. The worker must try to help family members come to terms with this, and to find ways of grieving the loss. However, the worker should explain that incremental changes are possible. For example, a client's son was a college graduate and had worked for a year as a teacher before developing full-blown schizophrenia. Since the onset of the disease, the son was unable to do what he used to do. The client was very upset about this loss and often asked if something could be done to help his son to "become a real person again." Indeed, he was so angry and unhappy that he had many conflicts with his wife and son. In my interviews with the client, I helped him express his feelings of loss and accept his son's rehabilitation potential.

MAJOR PERSPECTIVES ON WORKING WITH FAMILIES OF PERSONS SUFFERING FROM SERIOUS MENTAL ILLNESS

In the past thirty years, two major research and practice theories have been developed to understand the issues relating to families having a relative suffering from serious mental illness: (1) family burdens and (2) expressed emotions (EE). Generated from these two lines of research are intervention models and programs that attempt to tackle the issues confronted by family members.

Studies on Family Burdens

This area of research assumes that families do not "cause" mental illness in their relatives. Conversely, families suffer from burdens and poor physical and mental health as a result of caring continuously for their relatives with serious mental illness (Noh & Turner, 1987; Wong, 2000). Moreover, this line of studies assumes that family involvement plays an important role in successful rehabilitation. Specifically, family members provide resources and act as partners to formal mental health professionals in rendering support to their relatives. Some researchers even venture to suggest that professionals do not always understand the needs and issues faced by the client and that it is important for family members to form grassroots organizations to advocate their rights and redress the harmful effects of discrimination (Hatfield & Lefley, 1987).

Family burdens have been conveniently divided into categories of objective and subjective burdens (Noh & Turner, 1987). Objective burdens refer to practical difficulties faced by caregivers in the day-to-day care of their relatives with mental illness. Subjective burdens refer to psychological and social costs associated with the care of the relatives with mental illness.

Objective Burdens

Objective burdens include three categories of practical difficulties: understanding the disease, managing the symptoms, and coordinating therapy services. Three categories are outlined in the following paragraphs.

Lack of understanding of the cause of illness, of the treatments necessary, and of the mental health system. It is quite common to find that family members do not have adequate and correct information on the cause of mental illness and on the treatments available for their relative. Moreover, many families do not understand the types of services available and how to access those services. As a consequence, such families take a long time to reach formal psychiatric services for help and often seek other forms of therapy. For example, some families have arranged for their relatives to practice shamanism, to consult traditional Chinese doctors for herbal medicines, and to visit different Buddhist monks and Taoist priests for divine advice and interventions (Pearson, 1993). Due to a lack of information, family members may encourage participation in these alternative activities while their relative is still taking psychotropic medications prescribed by the psychiatrists, setting the illness sufferer up for potentially harmful side effects. Since not all therapy practices are successful, family members who participate in these different practices may invariably feel frustrated and disheartened when they do not see any change in their relative. In this case, the condition of their relative may continue to deteriorate, sometimes causing greater amounts of bizarre behaviors and excessive emotions. Thus, family members with adequate knowledge of the available and proven methods will experience less agony and frustration. In Hong Kong, studies conducted by Wong have revealed that caregivers expressed a lack of knowledge on the previously mentioned issues (Wong, 2000; Wong et al., 2003). Therefore, it is one of the primary duties of a mental health worker to enhance the knowledge of family members on the aforementioned issues.

Difficulty managing the problems of the relative with mental illness. Studies have suggested that family members, particularly the caregivers, complain of having difficulty managing drug compliance and medical follow-ups, bizarre behaviors, excessive and uncontrollable emotions, and negative symptoms of their relatives with mental illness. In one study, caregivers found negative symptoms such as "idling at home" and "lying in bed all the time" to be most burdensome (Wong, 2000). Managing positive symptoms relating to excessive and uncontrollable emotions and behaviors were the second most burdensome problem for caregivers (Wong, 2000). In Chinese culture, Confucian ethics espouse productivity and denounce inactivity. This cultural value may have some bearing on how caregivers perceive the negative symptoms manifested by their relatives. Indeed, caregivers who do not view these negative symptoms as resulting from the illness can become extremely frustrated. On the other hand, positive symptoms can be more easily recognized as part of the illness, and, therefore, may be a bit more tolerable than negative symptoms. It is important to educate caregivers to recognize and accept the positive and negative symptoms as part of illness, and they must also acquire knowledge and skills in handling these symptoms. Mental health workers should provide information and practical training sessions for family members to acquire knowledge and skills for managing the day-to-day care of their relatives. Family members in such situations have repeatedly expressed a need for practical advice on handling different management issues (Torrey, 1988).

Needing help in the coordination of services. The provision of psychiatric care involves such different departments as health care, social services, education, and vocational training, and involves different professionals such as psychiatrists, occupational therapists, psychologists, and social workers. Different operation units have their own sets of criteria and procedures for accepting service users. It is easy to appreciate the difficulties and confusion family members face when accessing the mental health care system. A mental health worker should provide a caregiver with information on the various psychiatric services available and should also help the caregiver connect to and secure the services for his or her relative.

Subjective Burdens

Studies have found that caregivers suffer from anxieties, frustrations, worries, guilt, grief, fear, and anger when caring for their relatives suffering from serious mental illness (Hatfield & Lefley, 1987; Wong, 2000). This gamut of emotions has contributed significantly to the poor mental health conditions found among caregivers. Subjective burden has been found to be a significant predictor of the mental health outcome of caregivers (Wong, 2000). In a comparison study conducted by myself and a team in Australia, results found that Hong Kong caregivers experienced a significantly higher level of subjective burden than their Australian counterparts (Wong, Jourbert, & Meadows, 2002). Social factors such as a lack of long-term residential facilities and psychiatric stigma as well as cultural factors such as the sense of familial responsibility among Chinese caregivers in Hong Kong have been used to explain the difference in the levels of subjective burden found in the two samples. One consequence of the prolonged exposure to subjective burdens is the high incidence of mental ill-health found among family members. In two studies, about one-third of the caregivers were shown to be at risk of having poor mental health (Wong, 2000; Wong et al., 2002). Thus, a mental health worker needs to give time and opportunity for a caregiver to ventilate his or her emotions. This is a necessary and important part of the counseling process because family members must learn to come to terms with the chronicity and irreversibility of the illness.

Social costs are being borne by caregivers with relatives suffering from chronic mental illness. Many studies have found that family members, particularly the caregivers, experience an increase in family conflicts, limited friendship and social life, financial difficulty, change in daily routines, etc. In the aforementioned comparative study, Hong Kong caregivers scored significantly higher in "social costs" than the Australian caregivers (Wong et al., 2002). Two cultural factors are used to explain these findings. First, Chinese parents still hold the belief that, as parents, they are forever responsible for taking care of their children, particularly the disabled ones. Second, Chinese parents who adhere strongly to the traditional views of the causation of mental illness may blame themselves for having "caused" the disease. In any case, these caregivers may want to compensate by spending a great deal of time taking care of their relatives with mental illness and ignoring their own physical and social needs. As a consequence they may experience mental health problems. Social costs are significantly related to mental health outcomes of caregivers (Wong, 2000). A mental health worker needs to spend time discussing this aspect of family burdens with the individual caregiver because (1) they need to learn to take good care of themselves and (2) they may become overly involved in the life of their relative and thus interfere with rehabilitation plans. However, the worker must be sensitive to the needs of the family members and help them gradually participate in ways that are best for their relative. The worker should not place blame or push the family members too quickly to loosen their responsibilities. Otherwise, they may reject the worker's involvement and may unintentionally sabotage the rehabilitation process.

Intervention Programs and Groups for Families Based on Family Burden Studies

Psychoeducation groups. This type of group aims at training family members to become long-term caregivers. It also helps prevent relapses in the relative with the illness. Essentially, it provides information on understanding mental illness, strategies to cope with psychotic symptoms, prevention of relapse, psychotropic drugs and side effects, social and vocational rehabilitation services, and the mental health of caregivers. In some groups, family members may also be given the opportunity to discuss and practice the previously mentioned skills. Other groups are simply run as lectures with questions and answers provided at the end of the group meetings. Experience has shown that family members had less burdens and better mental health after participating in the groups (Hatfield, 1998; Zhang, He, Gittelman, Wong, & Yan, 1998). However, several criticisms can be made about psychoeducation groups. First, many offer little opportunity for family members to discuss and deal with the psychological and social costs associated with the care of their relatives with mental illness. The group size is usually too large to facilitate sharing and mutual support. Second, although caregivers may have acquired more knowledge about mental illness and the skills needed to care for their relative, the groups do not give sufficient time to practice the skills.

Given these criticisms, it is useful to bear in mind the following points when organizing psychoeducation groups:

- Seminars of a larger group size can be organized to impart knowledge to family members; however, small groups of less than fifteen people should also be offered to deepen and personalize the knowledge gained through the seminars. In groups with fewer participants, family members feel more at ease to raise their concerns and questions. Moreover, workers have the time to address individual concerns and issues. Seminars without small groups risk arousing concerns and not giving enough time and space for family members to clarify the issues. Consequently, family members may become even more frustrated.
- Since a psychoeducation programs include medical information, it is quite common for a worker to invite a psychiatric nurse or a psychiatrist to deliver seminars. It is perfectly appropriate for these professionals to deliver the seminars; however, it is essential for them to present their ideas in nontechnical and user-friendly terms. Most family members will not understand and will feel threatened by technical medical terms. Moreover, the methods of some treatment options, such as psychiatric services, may be a bit complex for some family members, so it is necessary to design the contents so that family members can easily understand them. Generally speaking, the content should be simple, phrased in layman's terms, and be presented in a creative and interesting way.
- Enough group sessions must be provided for family members to have some practical knowledge and skills in managing the various difficulties they face when taking care of their relative. It is useful to include a few people who have had some successful experiences and ask them to share these experiences. However, it must be stressed that these are not skills-training groups and are not intended to train family members to acquire the management skills. Essentially, psychoeducation groups aim to provide information for family members. Family members who have gone through a psychoeducation group and are interested in pursuing skills training can be organized into a skills-training group.

Mutual-help groups. This type of group aims to provide family members with a place where they can vent their emotions and obtain support from fellow group members facing similar predicaments (Aristei & Finn, 2001). Mutual-help groups provide a place for members who have gone through difficulties in their caring roles to share their experiences with fellow group members. Indeed, some members may even act as role models for others in the group. This type of group also serves as a platform for family members to assert their rights by voicing their views and to find ways of improving psychiatric services for their relatives. Although the advantages of offering mutual-help groups are obvious, many obstacles can be encountered in establishing such a group. For example, in Hong Kong it is very difficult to recruit family members. Psychiatric stigma is so strong that some family members do not want to let others know that they have a relative suffering from serious mental illness. Another reason is that, due to busy lifestyles, some family members may not have time to join a group. Second, since this type of family group does not receive any financial support from the government, it does not have sufficient resources to support its operations. Last, it takes time to train leaders, and a long-term commitment among members is often lacking. To conclude, it is difficult to run a mutual-help group without funding from the government and without adequate support from the mental health professionals.

Given the previously mentioned difficulties, the following suggestions are helpful for organizing a mutual-aid group:

- The establishment of this type of group should involve at least one professional worker with past experience organizing a mutual-help group. The person can be a volunteer or a paid staff.
- The professional worker should assist the family members in setting up committees and should train committee members in their various roles. The professional worker should not, at any time, have the power to make decisions for the group. He or she should leave the decision making to the members.
- The professional worker should gradually pass the responsibilities of organizing and running the group on to the natural leaders who emerge during sessions. When the leaders have achieved independence, the worker should act as a consultant who provides advice only when asked. Another important function of

the professional is to provide encouragement and support for the leaders. In times of crises and conflicts, he or she may also act as a facilitator when requested to do so.

- Members of mutual-help groups should be aware of several on-going issues and of finding ways to resolve them, such as funding, having enough activities to maintain the vitality of the group, and maintaining harmony among committee and group members. It is necessary for members of the committee to continuously explore available resources that can fund recurrent expenses, because the group must structure regular and meaningful activities so that ordinary members can participate in them. Finally, members of the committee must be open and willing to forgo personal interests for the the common interests of the group. This requires members to constantly make reference to the common goals of the group.

Studies on Expressed Emotions

This line of studies was initiated by Brown, Birley, & Wing (1972) and Leff, Kuipers, Berkowitz, Eberlein-Vries, & Sturgeon (1982). Essentially, these studies focused on the examination of the dysfunctional communication patterns between family members and the relatives with serious mental illness. These dysfunctional communication patterns include critical comments, emotional overinvolvement, and hostility (Leff & Vaughn, 1985). *Critical comments* refer to "statements, which, by the manner in which they were expressed, constituted an unfavorable comment regarding the behavior or personality of the person to whom it was addressed" (p. 38), *hostility* denotes "generalized criticism and rejecting remarks made by family members toward the relatives with illness" (p. 41), and *emotional overinvolvement* concerns "behaviors such as exaggerated emotional response, self-sacrifice behavior, extreme over-protectiveness or preoccupation with patient's illness" (p. 45). Results repeatedly found that relatives whose family members had high scores in critical comments, hostility, and emotional overinvolvement (high expressed emotions—HEE) had a much greater chance of relapse than those with family members who scored low in these areas (low expressed emotions—LEE). Indeed, the difference was about 50 percent (HEE) and 20 percent (LEE) of relapse in the first year after having been discharged from the hospital (Mueser & Gingerich, 1994). However, recent findings suggest that cultural differences exist between the Western and Asian populations in their manifestations of expressed emotions. Among Asian cultures it is found that although family members exhibited a higher level of emotional overinvolvement than did Western families, it did not seem to account for the relapse and poor social functioning found among their relatives (Mueser, Bellack, Morrison, & Wixted, 1990). It has been argued, for example, that Chinese people, including the persons with mental illness, can tolerate a higher level of overinvolvement of family members. Indeed, it is culturally acceptable for parents to exhibit self-sacrificing and devoted behaviors. Thus, a relative with mental illness may not perceive such overinvolvement as an infringement of his or her personhood (Wong & Poon, 2002). However, emotional overinvolvement may affect the social life of a non-ill family member because he or she spends too much time taking care of his or her relative to participate in social and recreational activities.

Explanatory Models for the Relationship Between HEE and Relapse

Two models have been developed to explain the relationship between HEE and relapse in a person with mental illness: the attribution model and the interaction model. The *attribution model* suggests that how a family member perceives the behaviors and symptoms of the relative suffering from mental illness affects how he or she communicates with him or her. Family members who perceive their relative's behaviors and symptoms as negative and controllable tend to express negative comments and hostility toward their relative. Results of one study reveal that caregivers who perceive the behaviors of their relatives as controllable and negative exhibit more critical comments and hostility toward their relative (Wong & Poon, 2002). These relatives also had poorer scores in social functioning as well (Wong & Poon, 2002). However, one major drawback of this model is that it puts the blame for the problems onto the caregivers.

Other researchers have challenged this lopsided view and maintain that HEE is a result of an interaction and reciprocal relationship between the relative and the family members. This is referred to an *interaction model* of HEE (Kavanagh, 1992a,b). This model suggests that HEE is not solely a result of the family members' misunderstanding of the behavioral and emotional problems of the relative with the illness. In fact, it is an interaction between the two parties, and it is difficult to single out who is responsible for the development of HEE in a family. For example, a relative with severe positive and negative symptoms is unmotivated and has very poor self-care. Family members have repeatedly tried to help this relative improve his situation. However, due to the severity of his illness, his conditions remain the same. It is quite easy for family members, then, to become intolerable of his behaviors and start to criticize him. In turn, this relative reacts negatively to the criticisms and become argumentative. As a result, HEE may escalate. This example illustrates how both family members and the relative have contributed to HEE in the family, and that interventions should target at both parties. The interaction model is more often successful than the attribution model in understanding and dealing with the communication problems in HEE families.

Interventions for Reducing HEE in Families with Relatives Suffering from Schizophrenia

Studies on HEE have consistently demonstrated that families with HEE who went through communication-skills training showed marked reduction in expressed emotions and in the risk of relapse of the relative with serious mental illness, which was reduced by about 60 percent. Results compared favorably to the control groups, which showed only a 10 to 20 percent reduction in relapse rate (Palloon et al., 1982).

. Leff et al. (1982) and Falloon et al. (1982) are the earliest groups of therapists who adopted a family approach in working with families with HEE. The three major components in their work with families with HEE are (1) psychoeducation, (2) communication-skills training, and (3) problem-solving-skills training.

Psychoeducation. The main objectives of psychoeducation are to help family members understand and develop proper attitudes toward their relative with mental illness and to acquire basic information on the day-to-day management of their relative. It is quite customary to educate participants on the causes of mental illness, on the effects and side effects of medications, and on the relevant rehabilitation services available in the community. As well, it is essential to inform family members of the relationship between HEE and relapse. As part of psychoeducation, it is also useful to discuss the issues regarding relapse prevention.

Communication-skills training. This is an important component of the program and aims to help family members and clients develop better communication skills. Communication skills usually included in the program are:

- Expressing positive feelings and giving positive feedback
- Expressing expectations and setting rules
- Active listening
- Appropriately expressing negative emotions, anger, and disapproval

Several steps are involved in the process. First, family members and clients must jointly identify any communication problems. For example, in one of my family cases I videotaped a dialogue between the family members and the relative and reviewed the process with them. Throughout the review I pointed out their communication problems. I then discussed alternative and more appropriate communication skills, drawing their attention to how the new skills might make a difference in their lives. The last step involved having the families rehearse and practice the new skills during and between sessions.

Problem-solving skills training. The third component involves providing practical advice for handling the difficulties family members have in managing the day-to-day care of their relative with mental illness, including facilitating drug compliance, managing the excessive and fluctuated emotions, dealing with negative symptoms, etc. Since too many different types of management problems exist to be discussed in any one program, workers should consult participants before designing the content of this third component. Sufficient time should be given to participants to practice the various skills during and between sessions.

Although no standard format exists for this type of program, it can be run in a group format. Participants can be exclusively family members or can be multifamily members, including the relatives with mental illness. Moreover, problem solving can also be designed as a parallel group with several joint sessions being attended by family members and the relatives with the illness. Since family groups require members to share and practice communication and problem-solving skills, the size of a group should be about ten participants or about three to five families with an average of two to three members per family. Since the group may involve multiple families and may be with or without the ill relatives, it is better for this type of group to be co-led by two workers.

Criticisms of Expressed Emotions

Although EE can be explained in terms of an interaction model, HEE families may still perceive this negatively, thinking that they are somehow responsible for contributing to the problems and relapses of their relatives with serious mental illness. As a consequence, family members may either blame themselves or react strongly to this label. It is therefore important for a mental health worker to help family members understand the EE concept in a balanced light and encourage them to participate in a group. Second, this concept does not clearly emphasize the positive aspects of family communication and family resources. Although some family members have HEE, it should be recognized that family may have positive attributes and resources as well. Simply put, families should not be viewed exclusively as pathological. The third criticism is that cultural variations occur in terms of the manifestation of expressed emotions (Leff & Vaughn, 1985). As mentioned previously, Asian people have a high level of emotional overinvolvement. However, for Asians, this aspect does not correlate with relapse and social dysfunctions in a relative with serious mental illness. Indeed, it is advisable for the mental health worker to help family members develop their social lives.

GUIDELINES FOR WORKING WITH FAMILIES OF MENTALLY ILL PERSONS

Families should be regarded as partners.

Mental health workers should accept family members as partners and resources in the rehabilitation of a person with serious mental illness. This is theoretically and practically sound, because mental health professionals simply do not and cannot spend as much time and effort as can the family in helping the client with mental health problems. Indeed, family members often have a great deal more knowledge and resources than the professional expects. Mental health workers need to trust family members and include them as part of a treatment team. However, in many cases, this idea has been given only lip service. Family members simply do not receive the due respect they deserve from mental health workers.

Practical advice should be provided for family members.

Family members face a variety of problems in managing their relative with serious mental illness. They want to know the best ways of handling the various difficulties. Therefore, it is useful for mental health workers to provide as much practical advice as possible. Indeed, mental health workers need to equip themselves with a repertoire of strategies and skills in handling persons with serious mental illness.

Family members should be helped to express their emotions.

Since family members experience different emotions at various stages of their relative's mental illness, mental health workers should provide enough room and time for family members to fully express their emotions. Moreover, they should be prepared to face very negative emotions expressed by these family members. Understanding and acceptance are key to supporting these families. When family members have adequately expressed their emotions, they are then better able to accept the conditions and to start making constructive changes. In my clinical experiences, it is not uncommon to find family members having very negative emotions even after ten to twenty years. Indeed, they have not yet been helped to express their emotions. This is certainly psychologically unhealthy for family members and their relative.

Help family members attend to their own needs and to rebuild their social lives.

It can be counterproductive for family members to continue caring for their relatives when they are under stress, so it is necessary for family members to "recharge" their energy by taking a break from caring for their relative. Indeed, since many families have a tendency to become emotionally overinvolved, and since quite a few are at risk of developing poor mental health, they should be encouraged and helped to establish more fulfilling and interesting social lives.

Provide service options for family members.

At present, as indicated earlier in this chapter, few services catering to the needs of family members with a relative suffering from serious mental illness are available. Since a large number of mentally ill individuals live with their family, and some these family members have taken up the caring roles, the government has the responsibility to provide resources and funding to support these family members. In essence, if family members can adequately perform their caring roles, it may reduce the chance of their relative's relapse and consequently fewer hospitalizations will occur.

CASE ILLUSTRATION

Background

Lo was a thirty-two-year-old man with chronic schizophrenia and borderline intelligence. He lived with his family, which was comprised of a father (sixty-two years old), mother (fifty-eight years old), and two older sisters in a public housing estate. Lo was working at a sheltered workshop. His mother and one of his sisters attended our caregivers' support group. Lo's mother mentioned that her husband had retired and was rather uninvolved in the family affairs. He was very critical of Lo and would scold him for behaving inappropriately. Since Lo had developed the habit of picking up foods with his hands whenever and wherever he spotted them (on the table before dinner, in the street, etc.), his father refused to eat with him at mealtimes. Indeed, Lo's father would eat before the rest of the family. In Lo's mother's eyes, her husband was very distant and unsympathetic toward his son. Sometimes, Lo's father would complain to his wife, "Why don't you stop him from doing these embarrassing behaviors? He is a disgrace to the family." Out of anger and frustration, Lo's mother would argue with her husband, and as a result conflicts between the couple escalated.

Lo's mother was the main caregiver. She worked around her son's daily schedule. She was a part-time cleaner and claimed that she had to finish work by 4:00 p.m. As she said, "I have to be home by four p.m. because my son will be back at around four-thirty p.m." Further probing revealed that Lo had displayed some inappropriate sexual behavior toward his two sisters and that his mother felt that she had to be home to make sure that he would not do anything to them again. Besides work, Lo's mother spent almost all her time with her son and had not had a vacation for at least eight years. Her daughter mentioned, "My mother thinks that because of poor diet and a fall that happened during pregnancy she has brought mental illness to my brother."

Although one of the sisters was supportive and accepted her brother's behaviors, the other sister was afraid of him. In fact, this other sister was the victim of his sexual misbehavior. As Lo's mother said, "She [the other sister] came home very late in order to stay away from him as much as possible. She doesn't like him and wants to move out. I beg her not to. I don't want to see this family disintegrate." Indeed, it could be said that this sister was a bit hostile toward the brother.

Goals and Interventions

Besides helping Lo's family through the support group, I met with Lo's mother and sister to help them deal with some of their family problems. We identified the following goals:

1. Since Lo's mother was extremely stressed, we decided to provide her with as much time and opportunity for expression of her emotions as possible. Her daughter would also give her as much support as she could. Lo's mother was able to air out her feelings during the group sessions, and was also able to vent her feelings to me and to her daughter. Indeed, her daughter had become a very important support-ive network for her.

2. Lo's mother harbored a few misunderstandings about mental illness and believed that she had caused Lo to develop schizophrenia. Like-wise, Lo's father did not have sufficient understanding of Lo's illness and did not realize the detrimental effects of his communication on his son. I provided them with information on mental illness and the effects and side effects of medications. I told them that Lo's intelligence might have complicated the matter and his rehabilitation progress. Accord-ing to Lo's mother, although Lo's father was becoming a bit more toler-ant of Lo's behaviors because of counseling, he did not seem to be any friendlier or involved in Lo's life.

3. I interviewed the entire family, except the other sister (she never showed up). In the interviews I complimented them for keeping the family together and I let them express the difficulties they faced in the process. Each one of them, except Lo, was able to vent their frustra-tions. I tried to point out their strengths and how well they had coped with the difficulties. It turned out to be a good opportunity for the family to talk together (they had never done so before) and to better under-stand one another's views. As a result, they were able to appreciate one another's efforts and concerns. Moreover, the mother began to re-alize that other family members were concerned as well and that she

was not alone in the caring process. We also spent some time discussing how they could better manage Lo's behaviors, particularly during mealtimes and in public places.

4. I spent a bit of time with Lo's mother discussing her undue sacrifice for her son. Although I validated her efforts, I encouraged her to reestablish some social life and activities for herself. She began to make friends with other group members, and she eventually agreed to take a five-day vacation. This was a breakthrough for her and she started to realize that her son could be left temporarily in the hands of others. Moreover, since she had had a break and felt relaxed, she had re-energized herself. Indeed, she became much more happy than before.

This chapter has outlined two major areas of research in understanding and helping family members with a relative suffering from mental illness. Studies on family burdens help us understand the objective and subjective burdens and poor physical and mental health of family members who continuously provide care for the ill relative and the importance of providing psychoeducation and mutual-help groups for family members. Studies on expressed emotions have pointed out how dysfunctional communication patterns in a family may lead to a greater chance of relapse in the ill relative. Intervention programs that attempt to help the family members develop proper attitudes toward their relatives, acquire basic information on the day-to-day management of their relatives, improve communication skills, and enhance problem-solving skills are found to be useful. Indeed, it is necessary for mental health workers to see family members as partners and resources in the care of people with a serious mental illness.

Chapter 9

Handling Psychiatric Emergencies

INTRODUCTION

Psychiatric emergency refers to a situation in which a person is at risk because of intense personal distress, suicidal intentions, or self-neglect. Others in psychiatric emergency may behave in an aggressive manner, make threats and act violently (Atakan & Davies, 1997). These intense emotional and behavioral states are usually related to acute psychotic episodes, acute psychological crises stemming from life transitions, traumatic experiences, existential despair, routine problems in living, etc., and usually indicate the failure of the person to adopt his or her usual pattern of coping and use of a social network to circumscribe the crisis situation. As a consequence, psychiatric intervention is necessary. In Hong Kong, the official definition of psychiatric emergency is

> a condition under which a person's disturbance in thoughts, feelings or behaviors is to the extent of being out of control of him/herself, severely withdrawn, asocial, completely disoriented and out of touch with reality, jeopardizing his/her own health or seriously disturbing others, and is considered by the person him/herself, or by others, to require immediate outreaching service and psychiatric or other intervention (Social Welfare Department, 1999, p. 1).

ISSUES AND SERVICES REGARDING PSYCHIATRIC EMERGENCIES

Issues

In Hong Kong, the actual number of people needing intervention for psychiatric emergencies is unknown. Statistics provided by the Rehabilitation and Medical Social Services branch of the Social Welfare Department (Lau, 2001) on 1,190 cases handled by approved social workers between 1990 and 2000 suggest that the ratio of males and females needing psychiatric assessment was nearly the same. Thirty percent of the cases were unknown to the psychiatric system prior to the assessment, about 33 percent were actively receiving medical/psychiatric treatments, and about 36 percent had defaulted treatments. About half of the cases were under the age of forty, and about 36 percent were between the ages of forty-one and fifty. Finally, about 38 percent of the cases were compulsorily admitted and another 22 percent admitted themselves voluntarily to treatment. However, these figures did not tell much about the circumstances surrounding these psychiatric emergencies, nor did the figures disclose information about the diagnoses of the cases.

In another study, Stefanis, Rabe-Hesketh, Clarke, and Bebbington (1999) suggested that more than 49 percent of those using psychiatric emergency clinics were individuals with neurosis and major depression. Forty-seven percent had psychosis and manic-depression, and 40 percent had drug and alcohol problems. Among those who attended psychiatric emergency clinics, only 32 percent were acutely disturbed, and 17 percent exhibited unpredictable and violent behaviors. In Hong Kong, Chiu, Poon, Fong, & Tsoh (2000) analyzed 354 patients who had used the services of a community psychiatric treatment (CPT) team. The majority of the patients (about 72 percent) could be classified as having schizophrenia and delusional disorder. About 7.7 percent suffered from organic mental disorders and 5.7 percent from major depression. It is also revealed that about 21 percent had a past history of violence and about 14 percent had a recent episode of violence within the four weeks of the study. The majority of the individuals suffered from a psychotic or delusional disorder. In this sample, about 4.5 percent of patients had a history of attempted suicide and six people had attempted suicide in the four weeks prior to the study.

A study conducted by Lau (2001) on the decision made by approved social workers in Hong Kong to compulsorily admit a client for psychiatric assessment and treatment found four major personal risk factors leading to compulsory admission: the presence of active psychotic symptoms and of self-harm behaviors, the lack of insight into illness, and the loss of emotional control. The presence of a vulnerable individual (e.g., a child) and inadequate social support are two major environmental factors considered risks by the approved social workers in the assessment process. Way and Banks (2001) suggest that level of danger to self and others, severity of the psychosis, ability to care for self, impulse control, and severity of depression are major indicators for hospital admission. Indeed, the severity of the psychotic symptoms, possible danger to others or self, and lack of impulse control are the three major factors leading to hospitalization that have been consistently mentioned in the literature on psychiatric emergency. However, the availability or absence of social support is perceived as another important determinant of psychiatric admission among the approved social workers in Hong Kong.

Psychiatric Emergency Services

Different models are utilized for psychiatric emergencies, such as specialized psychiatric emergency services, mobile teams, and crisis residences. Many of these models are run concurrently.

Specialized Psychiatric Emergency Services

Psychiatric emergency services are hospital based, with special units established for handling such patients. In many ways, this is similar to an emergency department of a general hospital. Essentially, people with suspected psychiatric crises are sent to this unit for psychiatric assessment and observation by the personnel of a psychiatric team. Those who are suspected to be experiencing psychiatric crises will be detained for further observation. The service is round the clock. The advantages of a separate psychiatric emergency service include having a team of psychiatric professionals to assess and provide crisis management for people in psychiatric emergencies and having full-time service available twenty-four hours. Advocates of this service suggest that medical staff of the general hospital emergency unit may not have the expertise and skills to assess and manage a person in psychiatric crisis. However, the obvious disadvantages of the model are that it is more expensive to run a separate emergency service and that money spent on this service takes away from other psychiatric services. Another problem is that patients and families may feel stigmatized for being sent to such a "special" unit in a hospital.

In Hong Kong, no specialized psychiatric emergency services are available in hospitals and people in psychiatric crises must seek help from the Accident and Emergency Departments (AED) in the general hospitals. As soon as a patient is examined by a doctor at the AED, a psychiatrist may be called upon to conduct a more thorough psychiatric assessment of the individual. The person may then be asked to stay in the observation room of the hospital. However, no data is available regarding the profile of patients in psychiatric crisis who have used AED services in Hong Kong.

Mobile Crisis Teams

Mobile psychiatric crisis assessment and treatment teams have become an integral part of the mainstream psychiatric services in many countries. It is believed that such a service can prevent hospitalization and improve the well-being of mentally ill clients in the community (Guo, Biegel, Johnson, & Dyches, 2001). Recent studies using a quasi-experimental design and randomized trial have found that the availability of a community-based mobile crisis team resulted in a lower rate of hospitalization than did hospital-based interventions (Guo et al., 2001), in a greater symptom improvement, and in more patient satisfaction (Merson et al., 1992).

Three variations exist in mobile teams operating in different parts of the world (Allen, 2002). The first type is the psychiatric crisis management team that works on a round-the-clock basis, rendering assessment and treatment to suspected and known mentally ill clients in a crisis situation within the community. This team is usually comprised of professionals from various disciplines, including psychiatrists, nurses, psychologists, and social workers. In Hong Kong, some CPT teams adopt this psychiatric crisis management model. However, some do not run on a twenty-four hour basis, nor do they provide services seven days a week. The mobile crisis hotline and assessment team of the Social Welfare Department falls into this type of mobile service as well.

The second type of mobile team does not operate on a crisis management basis but emphasizes outreach and helping clients live independently in the community. Workers visit and render medical and psychosocial care to the clients regularly. This service may or may not be run for twenty-four hours and seven days a week.

The third type of mobile clinic provides medical treatment for the hard-to-reach clients (Allen, 2002). This service model has been used to work with the homeless, the elderly, and mentally ill substance abusers. In Hong Kong, community psychiatric nursing services fall into the second and sometimes third types of mobile team services.

Crisis Residence

Crisis residential service has become another component of psychiatric emergency service in the mental health care system. The main purpose of crisis residence is to provide an alternative to hospitalization for individuals experiencing a psychiatric crisis. It is hoped that people in psychiatric crises can have a temporary place for rest. This type of short-term, supportive-housing service is less restrictive, less stigmatizing, less traumatizing, and more normative than hospital services. Some of these residences are provided with professional staff, and others may use fellow consumers or volunteers to run the residence. Normally, an individual will stay in the residence for not more than two weeks and will be referred to another level of care or to return home. In Hong Kong, this type of crisis residence is nonexistent.

THERAPEUTIC FUNCTIONS OF PSYCHIATRIC CRISIS

Mental health workers generally find psychiatric emergencies stressful and difficult to handle. However, it is necessary to remember that psychiatric emergencies may have positive therapeutic functions for clients and for their families. To begin with, it is a time when the worker can openly express his or her concerns and to render practical help to the client. Indeed, crisis provides a good opportunity for the worker to build a close relationship with the client. Likewise, it is also a time for the worker to establish a relationship with the client's family members as well. Since it is not always possible for the worker to engage family members during "normal and quiet" moments, a psychiatric crisis provides the worker a chance to meet and establish rapport with the family members. Second, during a crisis situation, the client and his or her family members may be more willing to listen and work with the worker. Therefore, the worker can make use of the opportunity to educate family members on issues relating to mental illness, treatment, and relapse prevention. Finally, since a crisis usually implies a breakdown of the coping mechanisms of the client and of his or her family members in handling problems, a crisis provides an excellent opportunity for all family members to examine their coping mechanisms and to learn new and adaptive ones.

CRITICAL DECISIONS
IN PSYCHIATRIC EMERGENCIES

Three questions are crucial in psychiatric emergencies: (1) Is this a genuine psychiatric crisis? (2) Should this person be hospitalized? and (3) Should the police be called to help? (Lau, 2001). Affirmative answers to these questions lead to decisions and actions that are important to the lives of the individuals involved. The very first question (Is this a genuine psychiatric crisis?) is important to ask because not all psychiatric conditions are psychiatric crises. The definition of a psychiatric emergency was given in the beginning of the chapter.

An individual experiencing active symptoms of mental illness or relapse, such as persecutory delusions and severe depressed moods and self-neglect, but who does not constitute a possible danger to self or others is not considered as being in a psychiatric crisis that requires immediate intervention by the mental health professionals.

The second question (Should the person be hospitalized?) is a rather difficult decision to be made because any attempt to hospitalize or remove the person from his or her home can create tremendous anger and resentment in the person and in the family members. However, in some situations, this kind of decision is unavoidable. At least four conditions warrant a consideration to hospitalize or remove the person from the home environment: (1) the person poses a possible danger to self or others, (2) the person lacks a supportive network to closely monitor him or her, (3) the crisis is not likely to be resolved even with an increase in professional input or psychotropic medication, and (4) family emotions are escalating and the person is likely to respond negatively when unintentionally provoked by the family members. When hospitalization must occur, the mental health worker should discuss the decision with and explain the decision to the person and his or her family members. Only when this fails should the worker consider initiating involuntary admission for the client.

The third decision is an even harder one to be made by any mental health professional. The final question (Should the police be called to help?) will invariably evoke great emotion in the client and his or her family members. However, this decision is to be made when (1) danger to self or others exists, which includes potential harm to the worker; (2) the person has recently attempted to harm himself or herself or has recently acted violently toward others; and (3) the person's behaviors and emotions have become unpredictable. For example, people under the influence of alcohol or illicit drugs may act impulsively and aggressively. In those circumstances, the worker may need to consider calling the police for assistance. It is quite controversial as to whether the person should be forewarned or informed of this decision. In many instances, the conditions are so urgent that a forewarning is not considered or is deliberately unobserved in order to avoid provoking immediate retaliation from the client. However, when the client's emotions or mental conditions have stabilized, the worker should try to explain the decision to the client and his or her family members.

ASSESSING AND WORKING WITH INDIVIDUALS AT RISK FOR SUICIDE

Facts About Suicides in Hong Kong

In 2001, suicide ranked as the seventh leading cause of death in Hong Kong and contributed to about 3.1 percent of the total deaths (Hong Kong Jockey Club Centre for Suicide Research and Prevention, 2003). Although more females than males have attempted suicide, more males than females have died of suicide. Elderly suicide rates remain the highest among all age groups in Hong Kong. However, an increasing trend was found among middle-aged persons after the economic turmoil in 1997. In Hong Kong, jumping is the most common suicide method, probably due to its effectiveness and accessibility. Charcoal burning became the second most common suicide method used in Hong Kong in 2001, especially among the middle-aged persons. In the case of attempted suicide, the most common method used is poisoning (Hong Kong Jockey Club Centre for Suicide Research and Prevention, 2003).

Types of Suicidal Behaviors

At least four types of suicidal behaviors exist: completed suicide, attempted suicide, deliberate self-harm, and suicidal ideation (Tse, 2000) *Completed suicide* is self-explanatory. *Attempted suicide* refers to a potentially self-injurious behavior with a nonfatal outcome for which evidence (either explicit or implicit) that the person has intended to kill himself or herself exists. *Deliberate self-harm* is characterized by intentionally hurting oneself but with no intent to die (Pattison & Kahan, 1983). These individuals have a strong impulse to injure themselves, an increasing tension before the act, and an experience of either pleasure, gratification, or release at the time of committing the act. *Suicidal ideation* involves any self-reported thoughts of engaging in suicide-related behavior. All of these suicidal behaviors may potentially escalate into fatal acts that result in completed suicide. Thus, a mental health worker should take these suicidal behaviors seriously.

Risk Factors

Although suicidal risk assessment is one of the most important tasks in psychiatric emergency, efforts put toward identifying a specific set of risk factors to predict suicidal behaviors have not been very successful. It must be noted that any suicidal outcome involves a complex and interactive interplay of psychiatric, psychological, biological, and social factors (Maris, 1992). Indeed, the vulnerability-stress model can be used to conceptualize these various suicidal risk factors. Although a person may be biologically and psychologically vulnerable and be predisposed to commit suicide, it requires the presence of and an interaction with social and environmental factors for it to happen. On the clinical level, a mental health worker needs to carefully assess the various risk factors to determine the suicidal risk of an individual. In the literature, a number of risk factors have been identified as possible indicators of suicidal tendency. They are outlined in the following sections.

Biological Risk Factors

Diminished function of the neurotransmitter serotonin in the brain is said to be related to suicidal behaviors (Roy, 2001). One hypothesis about the relationship between serotonin and suicidal behaviors is that a lower concentration of serotonin reduces the ability of an individual to contain suicidal impulse (Roy, 2001). Specifically, a lower-than-normal concentration of serotonin in the cerebrospinal fluid is understood to be related to suicidal behaviors. Genetic studies also suggest that monozygotic twins have a significantly higher concordance for both suicide and attempted suicide than do dizygotic twins. Adoption studies also found similar results.

Studies on psychiatric morbidities have suggested that 90 percent or more of the individuals who committed suicide had one or more psychiatric disorders at the time of suicide (Roy, 2001). Harris and Barraclough (1997) conclude from a meta-analysis of studies on suicide that all psychiatric disorders, except mental retardation and dementia, cause an elevated risk of suicide. Among different types of mental disorders, depression (particularly major depression), alcoholism, schizophrenia, and personality disorders (especially borderline personality disorder), have been found to cause an increased rate of suicide (Roy, 2001). In his analysis, Roy (2001) suggests that depression is a comorbidity factor in other types of mental disorders such as alcoholism, paranoid schizophrenia and those with command hallucinations, and personality disorders. Since suicide is intimately related to depression, mental health workers must be careful when assessing people who have a mental disorder and have concurrent depressive symptoms.

Psychological Risk Factors

Certain personality factors are found to be related to suicidal behaviors, such as hopelessness, impulsivity, cognitive rigidity, and perfectionism. Hopelessness was identified by Beck, Rush, Shaw, and Emery (1979) as a major risk factor for suicide. It is believed that depressed people who express a sense of hopelessness pose a greater risk of suicide. However, recent studies have challenged this notion and suggest that hopelessness during a depressive episode was not predictive of suicide attempts. Rather, hopelessness as a premorbid personality factor seemed to predict future suicidal attempts (Young et al., 1996). Thus, people who have developed a strong sense of hopelessness as part of their personality makeups may have a high risk of suicide.

Another personality risk factor that is related to suicide is impulsivity. Whereas some studies suggest that people who committed suicide were more impulsive (e.g., Elliott, Pages, Russo, & Wilson, 1996), others have argued that suicide was related to mental illness and not to impulsivity (Tse, 2000). In other words, a person who is under the influence of persecutory delusions may act impulsively and commit suicide, therefore it is the disease that caused the suicide, not the impulsivity, which itself was just a product of the disease. Although no conclusive evidence on the relationship between impulsivity and suicide exists, a mental health worker should closely monitor individuals with poor impulse control and a previous history of suicide, particularly during times of personal distress.

Cognitive rigidity is another personality factor associated with suicidal behavior. People who are cognitively rigid think inflexibly, cannot think of alternatives, are poor in analytic and problem-solving skills, and are unable to examine consequences closely and carefully. In Beck et al. (1979), these individuals are said to be constantly engaging in dichotomous thinking and magnification. Thus, when they are confronted with stressful life circumstances they feel rather anxious and hopeless and cannot see any alternative to their problems. As a consequence, they may resort to suicide as the only solution to their problems.

Three types of perfectionism exist: other-oriented perfectionism, self-oriented perfectionism, and socially oriented perfectionism (Tse, 2000). People with other-oriented perfectionism expect others to meet their own standards, whereas those with self-oriented perfectionism make extremely high and unrealistic demands on themselves. Socially oriented perfectionists realize that external demands are unrealistic, but nevertheless feel that they have to meet those demands in order to gain social approval. Blatt (1995) found that socially oriented perfectionism was highly related to suicidal ideations. Since it can be frustrating to constantly try to meet others' increasing and high level of demands and expectations, individuals with this type of perfectionism may feel a lack of personal control and a sense of failure, anger, and hopelessness. As a consequence, they may develop suicidal ideations. In the assessment process, it is helpful for a mental health worker to gain some understanding of the cognitive flexibly and the perfectionist attitude of a client. This may be particularly useful for the worker to develop a longer-term intervention plan to help potential repeaters modify their cognitive rigidity and perfectionism.

Social Factors

Social isolation is a significant risk factor for suicide. Depressed people with a high degree of social isolation and poor social support have a greater chance of committing suicide than those who are not socially isolated (Maris, 1992). Perhaps, during times of distress, a person who is socially isolated does not have anyone to talk to and may engage continuously in negative thinking. As he or she becomes more depressed, his or her desire to commit suicide increases. On the other hand, another person who has a large social network is less likely to commit suicide because he or she uses the network for support during times of crisis (e.g., Nisbet, 1996).

Critical stressors in life are considered the "straw that breaks the camel's back" that trigger an individual to commit suicide. An extremely stressful life event can also drive a person to suicide. In order to ascertain whether a client will commit suicide, the mental health worker must ask the client or find out if he or she is currently facing any critical stressors in life (e.g., an unemployed person owing money to a loan shark).

Other Risk Factors

Previous suicide attempts. A person is more likely to attempt suicide if he or she has previously attempted to do so. Risk for suicide increases five- to sixfold if the person has attempted suicide previously (Maris, 1992). Moreover, the risk for a second attempt is highest within the three months after a first attempt. Some people may have multiple suicide attempts, and the worker should avoid viewing the cause as the person seeking attention from others. Although this may be the case, it is essential for us to treat any suicidal gestures or ideations seriously. The fact remains that the person may succeed in killing himself or herself, intentionally or not.

Concrete suicide plan. This is an important indicator for a person who wants to commit suicide. A concrete suicide plan includes (1) termination behaviors (e.g., writing a will, giving away valued possessions), (2) presence of lethal substances and objects at home (e.g., pills), and (3) a specific plan for committing suicide. The more concrete the suicide plan, the more committed the client is to killing himself or herself. Unfortunately, the more serious the client is about committing suicide, the more unlikely it is for him or her to disclose the plan to the worker. Therefore, the worker needs to slowly guide the client to give him or her the detailed information.

Chronic illness conditions. People who are depressed and suffer from a chronic condition are more likely to commit suicide than those without the condition (Yip & Tan, 1998). In Hong Kong, many elderly people who had committed suicide were found to have suffered from chronic illness (Yip & Tan, 1998).

Guidelines for Helping a Person with Suicidal Ideas

Assess the Seriousness of the Client's Suicidal Ideas

It is important to check whether the client has any concrete plan of suicide and to ascertain whether he or she thinks the method is going to end his or her life or if it is just a means of getting a message across to other people. If the person previously attempted suicide, it is useful to ask whether he or she is surprised to have survived and whether the action was impulsive or planned. Inexperienced workers are often quite worried about handling cases involving suicide. He or she may be fearful of leading a client to commit suicide by asking questions regarding his or her suicidal thoughts. The first lesson the worker should learn is that one cannot make another person commit suicide by asking him or her questions about suicide. On the other hand, if the worker does not ask the questions, he or she cannot find out whether the client may commit suicide. Chances are he or she may do it. If the worker can convey a sense of concern and care for the depressed person, it is easier to ask questions openly about suicide. The worker can explore any concrete plan of suicide and other risk factors present in the client. The worker must decide whether it is more appropriate for the client to be hospitalized than to stay in the community.

Help the Client Express His or Her Pent-Up Emotions

As mentioned previously, the worker needs to provide an atmosphere in which the client can express his or her pent-up emotions. Counseling skills such as empathy, active listening, and nonverbal communication have been found to be particularly useful to facilitate the expression of suicidal thoughts. However, it is not helpful to challenge or debate with the client whether committing suicide is right or wrong. Such a step might add shame and guilt to the client's already full bag of negative emotions. On the contrary, the focus is to help the client release his or her negative emotions.

Explore Alternatives with Client

Suicide is not a desirable option for solving problems. Indeed, no problems can be resolved through suicide. A severely depressed person is just lacking the capacity to think through the issues himself or herself. Although the worker may want to guide the client to explore the cons of committing suicide, he or she must also help the client find a reason to live. Once the client has found his or her reason, he or she may no longer contemplate suicide. For example, a severely depressed single mother may forgo the idea of committing suicide when she realizes that her children will become orphans if she dies.

As the worker guides the client to explore a reason to live, it is important for him or her to avoid creating shame and guilt in the client. The ultimate goal is to help the client have hope for the future. A way to help the client is to explain that he or she is currently trapped in the darkest moment in his or her life, and, although the client may not believe it, it will not get worse. Once he or she gets out of this darkest moment, he or she will be able to enjoy life again.

Remove Lethal Objects from the Client

Easy access to means of suicide is an important risk factor. It is important for the worker to ask the client if he or she has any accessible lethal objects. Should the client give an affirmative answer, the worker must negotiate with the client to remove these lethal objects. If this is impossible, the worker must consider other ways of preventing the client from completing the suicidal act (e.g., hospitalization).

Link the Client with a Support Network

It is paramount that a person who is suicidal is not left alone. In the interview, the worker needs to identify the client's confidants so that these people can be asked to "keep an eye" on the client before the next interview. The worker will need the client's consent to contact these confidants, and must ensure that the confidants can and know what to do if the client has suicidal thoughts again.

Establish a Contract with Client

If a depressed person who has vague suicidal thoughts does not need to be hospitalized, the worker should establish a contract with him or her. In the contract, it is necessary to spell out clearly what the client will do if his or her suicidal thoughts recur (e.g., calling the worker immediately, going immediately to a trusted neighbor's house). The contract must be as specific as possible (e.g., the name, telephone number, etc., of the person). It is useful for the worker to counter-check if the client has understood the terms in the contract and test his or her understanding and commitment to the contract. For example, after the worker has developed a contract with the client and before the end of the session, the worker may ask the client casually, "if you have suicidal thoughts again, who would you contact immediately?" If the client can answer, it means that he or she understands the plan and may have a greater chance of following the plan.

Document Every Decision Made During the Assessment and Intervention Process

Since suicide may have legal implications, it is necessary for the worker to record, in as much detail as possible, all the decisions involved in the assessment and intervention of the person with suicidal behaviors. It is important to document such details as clinical evidence for suicide, suicidal plan, and history of mental illness of the client, and it is also necessary to record the clinical decisions made by the worker and the rationales behind such decisions. If possible, documents such as any written contract and consent form should also be included. In the case of a verbal contract and consent, the worker should record this in the case file.

ASSESSING AND WORKING WITH PERSONS WITH AGGRESSIVE BEHAVIORS

Facts About Aggression and Violence

Aggression and violence are acts performed by an individual to self-protect or to dominate others, but always at the expense of the victim. Since violence occurs as a result of an increase in emotional pressure, the person who performs the violent behaviors, verbal and/or physical, may not be aware of the effect such behaviors have upon others and is unlikely to know when and how to stop his or her actions. The victim of such violence may experience physical and/or emotional pain. Although it is not easy to discern why a person performs violent behaviors, a reason for the behaviors always exists (Ward, 1995). For example, a young male client of mine with a head injury acted aggressively toward his father. On many occasions, it was difficult to discern the motives behind his aggressive and violent acts. Further exploration, however, revealed that the son had misinterpreted the father's tone of voice as being rejecting and hostile. As soon as he heard his father's voice, he tensed up and reacted at some point violently toward his father.

Cohen-Mansfield, Marx, and Rosenthal (1989) have classified aggression into four types: aggressive physical type (e.g., physical fighting and destroying items), aggressive verbal type (e.g., cursing and screaming), nonaggressive physical type (e.g., pacing), and nonaggressive verbal type (e.g., constant questioning). Others have differentiated aggression and violence in terms of their nature and suggest that aggression and violence can be premeditated or impulsive (e.g., Moyer, 1987). It has been suggested that the unpredictable nature of some violent behaviors is most threatening and fearful to family members and mental health workers during an emergency situation.

In Hong Kong, no known record exists of the number of aggressive and violent behaviors performed by people with psychiatric illnesses. However, the police classifications of homicide motives for 1,460 cases between 1976 and 1992 suggest that mental illness accounted for only 4 percent of the homicide cases in those twenty-six years (Broadhurst, 2005). More recent analysis has also suggested that mental disorders accounted for a very small proportion of the homicide cases between 1990 and 1996 (Broadhurst, 2005). It is generally agreed that the number of incidences of aggression and violence among people with mental illness is not any greater than in the general population. It should be stressed that most people who exhibit aggression and violence do not have a definable psychiatric illness, and most people with psychiatric illness do not act aggressively and violently.

Psychiatric Illness and Aggression and Violence

Various functions such as perception, judgment, and emotional state are involved in executing a human behavior. An act of violence undergoes similar cognitive and emotive processes. Some psychiatric illnesses can affect these processes, causing an individual to misperceive, make incorrect judgment, and express inappropriate emotions. As a consequence, the person may react with aggressive and violent behavior. It has been suggested that some types of mental disorders, such as antisocial personality disorder and paranoid schizophrenia, are more likely than others to be associated with aggressive and violent behaviors.

Psychosis

An individual in an acute psychotic state experiences various perceptual, cognitive, and emotional distortions. Such an individual is likely to make incorrect judgments about certain situations and people, and may respond aggressively and violently to outside conditions. Therefore, the chance of aggression and violence is increased among people experiencing an episode of acute psychosis. In addition, a client with paranoid schizophrenia who has developed a systematized delusional system against others is likely to misinterpret others' intents, thus inflicting aggression and violence onto others. Indeed, Taylor (1997) found that among psychotic forensic patients, delusions appear to have a direct role in the violent act performed by those patients. As a mental health worker, it is important to take note of the mental condition and verbal remarks of a client experiencing an acute phase of psychosis. Any escalating emotional and verbal responses made by this person toward others can be an indication that he or she may act aggressively or violently toward them. For example, a mental health worker should take note of the changes in delusional contents and the escalating emotions of a client with paranoid schizophrenia because, if the person feels increasingly mistreated by others, he or she may react aggressively and violently toward these individuals. In the case of a client with a fixed delusional target (usually one to a few people), it is important for the worker to keep track of any plan or action that the client may have toward the target, and, in some instances, may have to inform the target of any impending danger.

Mania

People who are manic but not psychotic show more anger and agitation than aggression and violence. In Cohen-Mansfield and colleagues' classification, this is referred to as a nonaggressive physical act that may not constitute violence (Cohen-Mansfield et al., 1989). However, since people in the manic state often present as irritable and perform socially unacceptable behaviors such as speaking loudly and acting intrusively, they are often misperceived by others as aggressive and even dangerous. Such behavior may provoke others' emotional reactions and result in a heated argument or a fight. However, people in the manic state do not normally act aggressively and violently. The mental health worker should try to help these individuals to calm down and avoid provoking them.

Case example. Mr. Roman was a thirty-three-year-old male client with manic depression. He came to my office one day demanding financial assistance from me. He appeared very agitated, spoke in a loud voice, and paced up and down my office room. I spoke to him in a soft and calm voice and invited him to share his concerns with me. When he became more composed, I escorted him to wash his face (this was done twice during the interview). Although I was on guard throughout the interview, I did not get a strong feeling that he was going to hurt me.

Head Trauma

People with head trauma, particularly frontal lobe injury, can become irritable and aggressive (Mezzich & Zimmer, 1990). These individuals have lost the ability to control themselves in provocative situations and react impulsively and aggressively. Since those with head injuries often have limited cognitive abilities, they have difficulties deriving and executing their problem-solving action plans. Out of frustration they may respond to the perceived threats with aggression and violence. Sometimes, these individuals may exhibit aggressive behaviors that are out of proportion to the situation. Moreover, they may at times act impulsively and unpredictably. Mental health workers and family members often find it difficult to manage individuals with a head trauma who act impulsively. Since the conditions of such individuals may not be amenable to medications and/or psychotherapy, some with very severe conditions may have to be put in institutions for close monitoring.

Case example. James, a young man in his early twenties, was involved in a car accident and suffered from a head injury. Since the head injury, his mother reported that James had repeatedly physically assaulted his father. Upon further probing, it was revealed that his father did not seem to understand the nature of James's illness, and constantly engaged in arguments with his son over minor issues happening at home. I tried to provide counseling for the father but found that he was unwilling to accept his son's situation. We tried to arrange a halfway house placement for James, but this failed because he punched another housemate on the second week of his trial stay. Eventually, James and his mother agreed to live in another house that the family owned, and he continued to receive day services from a nearby hospital.

Drug- and Alcohol-Related Aggression and Violence

People who are intoxicated with alcohol or drugs, especially cocaine or other stimulants, and those who are experiencing withdrawal, may act aggressively or violently even with the slightest provocation because they have difficulty restraining their impulses. Moreover, when intoxicated these individuals may misperceive the intentions of others, leading to a heated argument or a fight. It is important for the

workers to find ways of helping the person get sober and to avoid provoking them. Sometimes, outside assistance, such as from the police,
may be necessary in order to provide a safe environment for the clients, their family members, and for the workers involved.

Case example. John who was fifty years old had manic depression. His
wife called my colleague at work and said that John was drunk and threatened to kill her. My colleague called upon me to go with her to visit John's
family. At his front door, we could smell strong alcohol, and could hear John
screaming and swearing at his wife. We spoke to him at some length, but
found that his heightened emotions did not subside. Consequently, we felt
that we had to call the police to bring him to an emergency unit of the nearby
hospital.

Depression

Mental health workers may not be fully aware that people with depression can also exhibit aggression and violence. It is not uncommon to find that depressed persons commit homicide and suicide because they mistakenly believe that such an act can prevent someone
close to them from suffering. Moreover, mothers with severe post-
partum depression may attempt to kill their newborn babies. Therefore, mental health workers should be vigilant in assessing whether
the depressed individuals have any homicidal and suicidal tendency.

Risk Factors

Client's Mental Illness

As mentioned previously, several types of mental disorders may be
more closely related to aggression and violence than others. These include alcohol and drug abuse, antisocial personality, brain trauma,
and disorders with command auditory hallucinations to hurt others
and with persecutory delusions. These illnesses affect the perception,
judgment, and the consequential actions taken by the individuals concerned. However, it must be stressed that not every client with the
aforementioned disorders will be aggressive and violent. This serves
only as background information for further and more in-depth psychiatric assessment. This information also helps a worker to be more
careful in approaching a client with psychiatric illness during psychiatric emergencies. Nonetheless, several issues are important to re-

member when assessing the mental state of these individuals. First, during a psychiatric emergency, it is important to gauge the level of impulse control of the individual. An individual suffering from dementia, brain trauma, or who is under the influence of alcohol or drugs may have poor impulse control. Second, it is important to take note of the level of reality contact and the degree to which the individual believes in the command auditory hallucination or persecutory delusion. An individual under one of these two categories of psychotic influences may react strongly with aggression and violence toward others.

Past History of Violence

This is probably the most important predictor of potentially violent behavior. People who have a history of aggression and violence are more likely to repeat such behavior than those who do not have such a history. If possible, before entering a potentially violent situation, it is important for a mental health worker to secure information about the circumstances surrounding the person's violent behavior in the past: frequency, duration, intensity, the means used, intention, attribution of responsibility, and any criminal record that resulted. The worker should collect as much information as possible from the client's records and his or her family members and/or friends. However, it is necessary to point out that this individual does not necessarily act aggressively and violently. Assessment must take into consideration the personal and environmental factors that circumscribe any potentially violent situations.

Environmental Stressors and Triggers

It is not uncommon to find that some clients react aggressively and violently to certain environmental stressors or triggers. Lindenmayer, Crowner, and Cosgrove (2002) have suggested that the victims of violence perpetrated by people with mental disorders are most often people the mentally ill person knows, usually those family members who reside with them (Lindenmayer et al., 2002). This contrasts greatly with victims of violence in the general public who are usually attacked by strangers (Estroff, Swanson, Lachicotte, Swartz, & Bolduc, 1998). Lindenmayer et al. (2002) have argued that aggression and violence in persons with mental disorders arise mainly out of long-standing resentment and interpersonal conflicts between the individuals and their close associates. As such, it is important for the mental health workers to do two things: identify any family member who may be the potential victim of violence, and explore the interaction pattern between the victim and the perpetuator. This may facilitate some skills training that can help to address any underlying maladaptive interaction patterns between the persons and their close associates.

Guidelines for Working with a Person with Possible Aggressive and Violent Behaviors

Assess the seriousness of the client's aggression and violent behaviors.

It is important to find out whether the client has a definite target for aggression and violence, is under the influence of alcohol or drugs or psychotic experiences, has a sense of self-control, and/or possesses any means that can harm others. If the previous indicators are positive, and the client is experiencing an escalating emotional state, the worker should be acutely aware that a psychiatric crisis with potential aggression and violence is forthcoming. Some useful behavioral clues about impending violence include: (1) speech that is loud, threatening, and profane; (2) increased muscle tension; (3) hyperactivity (e.g., pacing); and (4) slamming doors or knocking over furniture.

. The worker should be prudent yet decisive in making decisions because he or she may need to solicit support from others as quickly as possible. In the case of a home visit, as a rule, two workers should visit the client together and a prior contingency plan should be made between the two workers. For example, when the client is becoming more and more agitated in the interview, one of the workers should solicit help from others, such as the police, while the other continues to engage the client in a conversation. Another point about home visit is that the workers should not enter the premises until they get a sense that it is safe to go inside. Otherwise, they should try to engage the client at the entrance. Even if they have decided to enter the premise, the workers should sit in a spot close to the exit and try not to let the client sit between the exit and themselves. Finally, the workers should inform their supervisor of their whereabouts and ask him or her to give one of them a call at a certain time (i.e., at the approximate time the interview should be finished).

In the case of an office interview, it is useful to have a buzzer or an alarm system in place so that the worker can call for help immediately. Similar to a home visit, the worker should sit close to the office door and invite a colleague to call near the end of an interview. In some practices, workers may actually open the office door during the interview. However, this should be used with discretion because it may infringe on the privacy of the client concerned.

Help the client express his or her anger and frustration.

Regardless of the truthfulness of the client's perception of the situation, it is important for the worker to provide an atmosphere in which the client can express his or her pent-up emotions. Counseling skills such as empathy, active listening, and nonverbal communication have been found to be particularly useful in this regard. It is important to remember that the worker is the "still center," allowing the client to express anger and frustration without feeling angry and threatened. When the worker is able to respond to the client's verbal threat calmly, his or her reactions would be less likely to provoke the client to become even more angry and frustrated. The worker should be observant when approaching the client, and should speak in a soft but firm tone of voice. He or she should keep a reasonable distance from the agitated and aggressive client. In addition, the worker should avoid arguing with the client about the validity of his or her perception and convey to the client that he or she is willing to listen to his or her concerns and is there to help. Finally, the elderly with dementia, who are confused and disoriented, can benefit from a calm and supportive tone, and need to be reassured that they are being placed in a safe and friendly environment.

Set limits firmly.

The worker needs to assure the client that he or she will do everything to help him or her control aggressive impulses, thus, the worker should set limits as to what the client can do when he or she is feeling angry and agitated. The worker must speak in a firm and calm manner, outlining what behaviors are tolerable and those that are intolerable. It is also important to let the client understand the possible consequences of his or her aggressive and violent behaviors.

Case example. Mr. Ling was a client of mine diagnosed with antisocial personality disorder. He had a long history of violent behavior beginning with childhood and had been in and out of the penal system all his life. In a particular episode, Mr. Ling accused other staff members of being unreasonable and was holding a chair in the air. His voice conveyed that he was becoming agitated and could act aggressively toward the staff. Since I had known him for quite some time and we had built a fairly good rapport, I spoke to him directly in a firm but concerned manner, saying that although I understood his unhappiness, his aggressive behaviors could not get him what he wanted. On the other hand, he might instead get himself into trouble again with the law. I told him that it was not appropriate for him to display anger and aggression toward the staff, but invited him to express his concerns calmly to them. Moreover, I assured him that I would do everything I could to help bring his concerns to the attention of the appropriate authority. In this instance, rapport that was built in the past and the firm but supportive tone helped prevent what could have been another episode of violence.

Provide drug treatment.

Drug treatment may be necessary for some clients who are extremely agitated and do not seem to benefit from other means of treatment. Likewise, physical restraint may be a realistic option for the few clients who are severely disturbed and cannot be controlled through other means. As a mental health worker, it is important to constantly keep in mind that the least restrictive measures possible should be used to manage persons with psychiatric disturbances. However, when a client's behavior affects the life of another person, no alternative exists but to adopt more restrictive measures. In such circumstances, a mental health worker should consult the medical teams and devise the most appropriate measure for the client.

Document everything.

Thorough documentation is important for handling psychiatric clients with violent behaviors. This is particularly crucial for procedures involving seclusion and restraint. Since any of these handlings may have legal implications, it is necessary for the worker to record, in as great detail as possible, all the decisions involved in the assessment and intervention of a person with aggressive and violent behavior. It is important to document clinical evidence pertaining to symptoms and circumstances leading to the decisions made, and it is also necessary to record those decisions made and the rationales behind the decisions. These decisions should have also taken into account a risk-benefit analysis. If possible, documents such as the written contract and the consent form should also be included in the file. In the case of a verbal contract and consent, the worker should record this in the case file.

GUIDELINES FOR WORKING WITH FAMILIES OF PERSONS IN PSYCHIATRIC CRISIS

Be calm and supportive.

In emergency situations such as violent outbursts, family members can become rather emotional and may feel helpless. Many do not know what to do and are glad that professionals are there to help. A mental health worker who appears calm and supportive is very reassuring to family members. In some cases, family members are able to devise strategies to handle the crisis once they feel that they are being supported. Indeed, it is important for the worker to help family members develop and utilize their own resources to handle psychiatric emergencies as much as possible. Unless family members can establish a sense of efficacy, they are very likely to feel powerless, and very unlikely to be able to handle such a psychiatric crisis independently in the future.

Decide whether to involve both family members and client in the interview.

If a family member, relative, or friend is present at a crisis situation, it is essential for the worker to decide early in the assessment process whether to include the family member in the interview with the client. Sometimes, a family member, relative, or friend may be the source of agitation and the target of aggression and should be interviewed separately. If two workers are present, one should interview the client and the other should interview the family member. However, the client should always be the major focus of assessment and attention should be devoted first to building rapport and understanding with him or her. Some family members may take over the conversation, in which case the worker should skillfully shift the focus back to the client.

Help family members express emotions during and after the crisis.

It is important for the worker to try to understand the views shared by family members concerning the aggressive and violent behavior of the client. As mentioned previously, family members feel emotional and helpless and that they need to be heard as well. Clinical experience suggests that unless family members are able to express and work through their fear, anger, helplessness, and other emotions, they may not be able to work constructively to help their relative manage his or her aggressive and violent behavior.

Assess whether it is necessary to temporarily separate the client from family members.

At times, when the worker is unsure of the potential violence of the client, and feels it may not be safe for other family members to live with the client, he or she must make a decision to temporarily separate the client from other family members. If possible, it is always preferable to involve the client in this decision, otherwise, he or she may feel betrayed by the family members and may become unhappy with them. A mental health worker should actively help the family members explore temporary alternative accommodations for the client.

Help family members develop a contingency plan for managing the crisis.

Should the client be regarded as safe to live at home after a physical or verbal outburst, it is useful to develop a contingency plan with the family and the client. If the impulse of violence returns, the client and/or the family members should call a CPT team (or similar service if it is available), the police, or bring the person to an emergency department of a nearby hospital. Moreover, the worker should inform the family that he or she will phone or visit the family at a specified date and time to see if the family needs further assistance. Finally, the worker should provide the family with contacts should a similar crisis occur.

CASE ILLUSTRATIONS

A Client with Suicidal Ideation

Mandy was a twenty-eight-year-old college graduate who was diagnosed as having major depression. Upon her separation from her boyfriend and the death of her mother, she became severely depressed. Her father died when she was a child, and her other relatives were distant. Socially, Mandy had a number of friends before the illness. However, as she withdrew, she stopped contacting them. She had only a few friends who still kept in contact with her over the phone. Although she and her boyfriend had ended their relationship, Mandy still saw her boyfriend occasionally and had the thought that he might one day change his mind. Mandy worked as a clerk in a government office.

I saw Mandy for about three months after her second admission to the hospital. She tried to commit suicide with an overdose but failed in the attempt. This incident was preceded by the news that her ex-boyfriend was getting married soon. Throughout the sessions, Mandy struck me as an individual who was rigid in thinking and became upset rather easily. If and when she encountered something that did not please her, she would become emotional and sometimes resort to inflicting self-harm or attempted suicide. She mentioned in one interview that as a high school student she had slashed her wrists a few times because her teachers and schoolmates did something that upset her.

Mandy called me one afternoon and spoke in a very shaky and low voice. She mentioned that her boyfriend's wedding was coming soon and that she could not bear to see him marry another girl. Although she knew that the day would come, she could not accept it. She said she had a strong impulse to end her life and didn't know what to do. While she was talking to me on the phone she broke down in tears. I was very worried because she bore a number of suicidal risk factors. These included a recent history of suicide, a psychiatric illness of depression, cognitive rigidity, social isolation, and a critical stressor that was linked to a recent suicide attempt.

A colleague and I visited her immediately. During the visit, we encouraged her to express her unhappiness and frustrations. Although she remained rather emotional, I asked her if she still had a strong urge to kill herself and whether she had any plan to do so. She said she had a bottle of pills with her and that she had had the thought of taking all of them. She did not see any reason to live, saying, "He deserted me and I wanted him to regret it for the rest of his life." We discussed hospitalization and she refused. I asked her how she had been taking care of herself and she replied by saying that she had not been eating much in the past few days and that she had not been sleeping well. She kept crying and repeatedly said she didn't know what to do. I remained as composed as I could and showed her my emotional support. We also explored whether anyone in her social network could provide her with emotional and instrumental support. Even though she could name a few persons, I did not feel that these individuals could provide her the support she needed. Since she kept saying that she did not know what to do, it struck me that she was ambivalent about killing herself. I had the feeling that she still wanted to do everything she could to save the relationship. Since I did not think this was a realistic goal, I found it inappropriate to discuss this with her. On the other hand, I just mentioned that she might need some time and a clear mind to think through the issues that bothered her and that I would be willing to be her sounding board in the future. I raised the issue of hospitalization with her again and suggested that she needed a good sleep and some time to calm herself down. She finally agreed to go to the AED with me.

A Client with Aggression and Violent Behavior

Mr. Luk was a sixty-year-old man who was diagnosed as having personality disorder of an unclear specification. He was referred to our halfway house after a hospital stay for about nine months. He was admitted to the hospital upon exhibiting an aggressive outburst toward his wife and two adult daughters. The referral note described Mr. Luk as someone who had difficulty controlling his temper and who potentially could act aggressively toward others. Indeed, one daughter was badly injured during one incident and had to be hospitalized for a few days. Since the daughters and the wife were rather frightened of him, they did not want him to return home immediately upon discharge.

In my interviews with his daughters and his wife, they described Mr. Luk as someone who always had a very bad temper. He would speak in a coarse voice even with the slightest provocation. He spoke in such a way that people around him became very frightened. However, he had never had any physical outburst until the incident with his daughter happened. Throughout the years, the daughters and the wife had maintained very minimal contact with him (they lived together in two separate but adjacent units of a public housing estate). The incident of attack was preceded by an unreasonable demand Mr. Luk made on his wife and the daughters who were present made an angry remark toward the father. Consequently, it escalated into a physical outburst by Mr. Luk.

When I interviewed Mr. Luk, he was rather evasive about the incident. However, I got the feeling that Mr. Luk felt sorry for what he had done to his daughter, and did not want to be put in the hospital again. Initially, he was trying very hard to control his temper, but kept demanding that I let him return to his housing unit. His temper became more apparent when we refused to let him return home immediately. I found that he had not been putting any genuine effort into participating in the family interviews, and his daughters and wife still did not feel comfortable about having him back home. It came to a point when an open communication among the two parties was needed and another family interview was therefore arranged. During one session, Mr. Luk appeared rather angry and hostile toward his daughters, and mentioned that they should not have asked me to be the mediator (i.e., an outsider should not be involved in their family affair). As he pounded his hands on the table a few times, I told him firmly that although I could see why he was very angry and frustrated, he should control his temper. I told him that his family and I were concerned about him and wanted him to return home as soon as possible, but his temper was so great and uncontrollable that both the family and I did not feel comfortable letting him return home. He became extremely angry and swore at me. I felt that I needed to set limits with him and told him that should he continue to behave in this manner, I would make him leave the room and cool himself down. As soon as he heard this he hit the table again and left the room. Although I did not perceive him as highly aggressive during that moment, Mr. Luk did have a number of risk factors. These included a recent history of aggression, an object of aggression (daughters), and environmental triggers (e.g., interpersonal conflicts with his wife and daughter).

After about five minutes, as I continued my interview with the two daughters, Mr. Luk came back to the office and became more settled. I encouraged him to express his frustrations and his desire to return home. I also helped his daughters express their concerns. I stressed that everyone in the family wanted him to return home, but he had to work hard to control his temper. This therapy session was a very important step for the family because, for the first time, the daughters were able to openly and fully express their concerns about their father's outbursts and about how much they cared for him, but were also afraid of him. Since that interview, Mr. Luk was more genuine in his attempt to learn ways of handling his temper outbursts. After nine months, he returned home to live.

This chapter has highlighted the assessment and intervention guidelines and skills for working with clients who are at risk of suicide and with those with aggressive behavior. When making an assessment of people who are at risk of suicide, it is necessary to examine the biological, psychological, and social risk factors and to assess the seriousness of the client's suicidal ideas. For a client with aggressive and violent tendencies it is essential to look at his or her risk factors and environmental stressors and triggers. Finally, mental health workers should take note of the guidelines for working with families of persons in psychiatric crisis.

Appendix I

Life Skills Assessment

In each of the following eight components (a through h), seven overt behavioral items are listed. If the person being assessed can perform the task completely on his or her own, he or she receives two points. One point is given for item(s) that can be done only partially or under supervision, and zero points are given if the person is not able to perform the task under any circumstances. Overall performance of each component is calculated by adding the points scored in each item. (0 = by observation; A = from assessment)

a.	Financial management	O	Able to use banking services (e.g., money deposit, safety box, cash machine)	_____
		O	Spends money based on basic living needs	_____
		O	Keeps money in a safe place	_____
		O	Has an idea of market prizes and able to use money according to his or her own financial situation	_____
		O/A	Able to make budget based on expenses	_____
		O/A	Knows how to plan and share expenses with family members/others	_____
		O/A	Knows what to do with surplus	_____
			Total	_____
b.	Self-care	O	Able to maintain basic body cleanliness (e.g., wash hair, take bath, wash face, brush teeth, etc.)	_____
		O	Able to maintain personal grooming (e.g., cut hair, wear clean clothing)	_____

		O	Wears clothing that is appropriate for weather	_____
		O	Aware of proper food to eat	_____
		O	Able to make an appropriate daily routine schedule (e.g., gets up and goes to bed on time, regular meal time with appropriate diet)	_____
		O	Washes and puts away clothing regularly	_____
		O	Able to make bed and keep personal area tidy	_____
			Total	_____
c.	Personal mental health	A	Has knowledge about the mental illness he or she is suffering from	_____
		O/A	Able to seek help when not feeling well (e.g., seeks help from a doctor, social worker, family members, staff, etc.)	_____
		O/A	Able to manage the effect of residual symptoms on daily living	_____
		A	Aware of his or her chance of rehabilitation	_____
		O/A	Aware and able to manage relapse symptoms	_____
		O/A	Understands and knows how to exercise patients' rights	_____
		O/A	Understands the physical impact of his or her mental illness	_____
			Total	_____
d.	Problem-solving ability	O/A	Able to work out the contributing factor(s) or cause(s) of issues/problems	_____
		O/A	Able to understand an issue or problem from different perspectives	_____
		O/A	Able to integrate and sum up different opinions, then make judgment and choices	_____
		O/A	Able to identify and use appropriate resources when dealing with a problem	_____

	O/A	Able to work with others in discussing and solving a problem	_____
	O/A	Able to learn how to solve a problem from experience	_____
	O/A	Able to actively face and deal with arguments or conflicts	_____
		Total	_____
e. Use of community resources	O	Has knowledge about the nearby roads and environment	_____
	O	Able to use public or private medical services independently	_____
	O	Able to use facilities for daily provisions (e.g., supermarkets, corner stores, pharmacies)	_____
	O/A	Able to make use of various public facilities independently (e.g., post office, bank)	_____
	O	Able to use various common public transports (e.g. bus, subway, train, ferry)	_____
	O	Able to make use of resources in various major government departments	_____
	O/A	Able to make use of municipal facilities independently (e.g., public parks, libraries, etc.)	_____
		Total	_____
f. Social skills	O	Exhibits age-appropriate behavior	_____
	O	Possesses and exhibits appropriate social etiquette in public places	_____
	O	Able to express own opinions and requests (using the right words of expression)	_____
	O	Able to respond appropriately to what other people say (including verbal and nonverbal expressions)	_____
	O	Able to control and express emotions and feelings	_____

		O	Able to relate harmoniously with others	_____
		O	Able to understand his or her own roles and what is expected of him or her in various institutions (e.g., family, work-place, residence)	_____
			Total	_____
g.	Medication habit	O	Understands and complies to instructions on the medicine package	_____
		A	Accepts medication	_____
		O	Takes accurate dosage of medicine	_____
		O	Knows the names of medicines	_____
		O	Stores medicine in a safe place (e.g., in a fixed and dry place, in the fridge when necessary)	_____
		O/A	Understands and knows how to manage the side effects of medicine	_____
		O	Counts and makes sure the correct amount of medicine is given after follow-up consultation	_____
			Total	_____
h.	Work	O/A	Understands the need to work	_____
		O/A	Has reasonable expectations regarding work	_____
		O/A	Has knowledge on how to seek a job	_____
		A	Is equipped with interviewing skills	_____
		O	Has good work habits	_____
		A	Knows how to relate with colleagues	_____
		O/A	Knows his or her labor rights	_____
			Total	_____

Appendix II

Self-Reward Exercise

Goal	Indicator of success	Personal reward

Appendix III

Physiological Symptom Checklist

	Not at all	Occasionally	Sometimes	Always
Shortness of breath (dysnea or smothering sensation)				
Choking				
Palpitations or accelerated heart rate (tachycardia)				
Chest pain or discomfort				
Sweating				
Dizziness, unsteady feelings, or faintness				
Nausea or abdominal distress				
Feelings of unreality (depersonalization or derealization)				
Numbness or tingling sensations (paresthesia), usually in the fingers, toes, or lips				
Flushes (hot flashes) or chills				
Others:				
Others:				
Others:				

Source: Adapted from Peurifoy, R. Z. (1995).

References

Allen, M. H. (Ed.) (2002). *Review of psychiatry,* Volume 21, *Emergency psychiatry.* Washington, DC: American Psychiatric Press.

American Psychiatric Association (2000). *Diagnostic and statistical manual of mental disorders,* Fourth edition, text revision. Washington, DC: American Psychiatric Association.

Aristei, M. & Finn, L. "Grow—A mutual help group for psychologically troubled people." Interview by N. Swan. *The Health Report,* Radio National, November 5, 2001. Transcript available at <http://www.abc.net.au/rn/talks/8.30/helthrpt/stories/s409316.htm>.

Atakan, Z. & Davies, T. (1997). Mental health emergency. *British Medical Journal, 314,* 1740-1742.

Australian Health Ministers (1992). *National Mental Health Policy.* Canberra: Australian Government Publishing Service.

Beck, A. T. (1979). *Cognitive therapy and the emotional disorders.* Boston: Meridian.

Beck, A. T., Emery, G., & Greenberg, R. L. (1985). *Anxiety disorders and phobias: A cognitive perspective.* New York: Basic Books.

Beck, A. T., Freeman, A., Davis, D. D., Arntz, A., Beck, J. S., Butler, A., Fleming, B., Fusco, G., Morrison, A., Padesky, C. A., Pretzer, J., Renton, J., & Simon, K. M. (1990). *Cognitive therapy of personality disorders.* New York: Guilford Press.

Beck, A. T., Rush, A. J., Shaw, B. F., & Emery, G. (1979). *Cognitive therapy of depression.* New York: Guilford Press.

Beck, J. S. (1995). *Cognitive therapy: Basics and beyond.* New York: Guilford Press.

Bentley, K. J. (1998). Psychopharmacological treatment of schizophrenia: What social workers need to know. *Research on Social Work Practice, 8*(4), 384-405.

Bernheim, K. F. & Lehman, A. F. (1985). *Working with families of the mentally ill.* New York: W.W. Norton & Company.

Blatt, S. (1995). The destructiveness of perfectionism: Implications for the treatment of depression. *American Psychologist, 50*(12), 1003-1020.

Bridges, K., Huxley, P., & Oliver, J. (1994). Psychiatric rehabilitation: Redefined for the 1990s. *The International Journal of Social Psychiatry, 40*(1), 1-16.

Broadhurst, R. D. (2005). Crime trends in Hong Kong. In R. Estes (Ed.), *Social development indicators for Hong Kong: The unfinished agenda* (pp. 185-192). New York: Oxford University Press.

Brown, G. W., Birley, J. L. T., & Wing, J. K. (1972). Influence of family life on the course of schizophrenic disorder: A replication. *British Journal of Psychiatry, 121,* 241-258.

Chen, C. N., Wong, J., Lee, N., Chan-Ho, M. W., Lau, T. F. J., & Fung, M. (1993). The Shatin Community Mental Health Survey in Hong Kong. *Archives of General Psychiatry, 50,* 125-133.

Cheung, H. K. (2001). A 2-year prospective study of patients from Castle Peak Hospital discharged to the first long-stay care home in Hong Kong. *Hong Kong Journal of Psychiatry, 11*(2), 1-12.

Chinman, M., Weingarten, R., Stayner, D., & Davidson, L. (2001). Chronicity reconsidered: Improving person-environment fit through a consumer-run service. *Community Mental Health Journal, 37*(3), 215-229.

Chiu, S. N., Poon, T. K., Fong, S. Y., & Tsoh, M. Y. (2000). A review of 354 outreach patients of the Kwai Chung Hospital Community Psychiatric Team. *Hong Kong Journal of Psychiatry, 10*(3), 6-13.

Cohen, S. & Wills, T. A. (1985). Stress, social support, and the buffering hypothesis. *Psychological Bulletin, 98*(2), 310-357.

Cohen-Mansfield, J., Marx, M. S., & Rosenthal, A. S. (1989). A description of agitation in a nursing home. *Journals of Gerontology, 44*(3), M77-M84.

Cook, J. A., & Razzano, L. (2000). Vocational rehabilitation for persons with schizophrenia: Recent research and implications for practice. *Schizophrenia Bulletin, 26*(1), 87-104.

Cowger, C. D. (1992). Assessment of client strengths. In D. Saleebey (Ed.), *The Strengths Perspective in Social Work Practice* (pp. 47-139). New York: Longman.

Diziegielewski, S. F. & Leon, A. M. (1998). Psychopharmacological treatment of major depression. *Research on Social Work Practice, 8*(4), 475-490.

Elliot, A. J., Pages, K. P., Russo, J., & Wilson, L. G. (1996). A profile of medically serious suicide attempts. *Journal of Clinical Psychiatry, 57*(12), 567-571.

Ellis, A. (1986). Rational-emotion therapy. In I. L. Kutash & A. Wolf (Eds.), *Psychotherapist's casebook* (pp. 277-287). New York: Springer.

Ellis, A. (1993). Reflection on rational-emotion therapy. *Journal of Consulting and Clinical Psychology, 61*(2), 199-202.

Estroff, S. E., Swanson, J. W., Lachicotte, W. S., Swartz, M., Bolduc, M. (1998). Risk reconsidered: Targets of violence in the social networks of people with serious psychiatric disorders. *Social Psychiatry and Psychiatric Epidemiology, 33* (Suppl. 1), S95-S101.

Falloon, I. R. H., Boyd, J. L., McGill, C. W., Ranzani, J., Moss, H. B., Gilderman, A. M. (1982). Family management in the prevention of exacerbation of schizophrenia: A controlled study. *New England Journal of Medicine, 306,* 1437-1440.

Falloon, I. R. H., Boyd, J. L., McGill, C. W., Strang, J. S., & Moss, H. B. (1981). Family management training in the community care of schizophrenia. In M. J. Goldstein (Ed.), *New developments in interventions with families of schizo-*

phrenics: New directions for mental health services, (Vol. 12, pp. 61-78). San Francisco: Jossey-Bass.

Falloon, I. R. H., Mueser, K., Gingerich, S., Rappaport, S., McGill, C., & Hole, V. (1988). *Behavioural family therapy: A workbook.* Buckingham, England: Buckingham Mental Health Services.

Gilbert, P. (2000). *Counselling for depression.* London: Sage Publications.

Glasser, W. (1984). *Control theory: A new explanation of how we control our lives.* New York: Harper & Row.

Gotlib, I. H. & Colby, C. A. (1987). *Treatment of depression: An interpersonal systems approach.* New York: Pergamon Press.

Gotlib, I. H. & Hammen, C. L. (Eds.) (2002). *Handbook of depression.* New York: Guilford Press.

Guo, S., Biegel, D. E., Johnson, J. A., & Dyches, H. (2001). Assessing the impact of community-based mobile crisis services on preventing hospitalization. *Psychiatric Services, 52*(2), 223-228.

Harris, E. C. & Barraclough, B. (1997). Suicide as an outcome for mental disorders. A meta-analysis. *British Journal of Psychiatry, 170,* 205-228.

Hatfield, A. B. (1998). Issues in psychoeducation for families of the mentally ill. *International Journal of Mental Health, 17*(1), 48-64.

Hatfield, A. B. & Lefley, H. P. (1987). *Families of the mentally ill: Coping and adaptation.* New York: Guilford Press.

Hatfield, A. B. & Lefley, H. P. (1993). *Surviving mental illness: Stress, coping, and adaptation.* New York: Guilford Press.

Health and Welfare Bureau (1999). *Hong Kong Rehabilitation Programme Plan Review (1998-99 to 2002-03): Towards a New Rehabilitation Era.* Hong Kong: Government Printer.

Hellewell, J. S. E. (2002). Patients' subjective experiences of antipsychotics: Clinical relevance. *CNS Drugs, 16*(7), 457-471.

Hersen, M., Bellack, A. S., & Himmelhoch, J. M. (1982). Skills training with unipolar depressed women. In James P. Curran & Peter M. Monti (Eds.), *Social skills training: A practical handbook for assessment and treatment* (pp. 159-185). New York: Guilford Press.

Hong Kong Council of Social Services & MHAHK (1996). *Public attitudes toward mental health problems and mental patients in Hong Kong.* Hong Kong: Hong Kong Council of Social Services.

Hong Kong Council of Social Services & MHAHK (1997). *Public attitudes toward mental health problems and mental patients in Hong Kong: A follow-up study over two years.* Hong Kong: Hong Kong Council of Social Services.

Hong Kong Jockey Club Centre for Suicide Research and Prevention. (2003). Suicide in Hong Kong. Available online at: <http://csrp.hku.hk/render1.php?template=a&content=content/a_aboutsuicide_suicideinhongkong.html>.

Intagliata, J. (1982). Improving the quality of community care for the chronically disabled: The role of case management. *Schizophrenia Bulletin, 8*(4), 655-674.

Kavanagh D. J. (1992a). Recent developments in expressed emotion and schizophrenia. *British Journal of Psychiatry, 160,* 601-620.

Kavanagh, D. J. (Ed.) (1992b). *Schizophrenia: An overview and practical handbook.* London: Chapman & Hall.

Kendall, P. C. & Hammen, C. (1995). *Abnormal psychology.* New Jersey: Houghton Mifflin.

Lau, D. Y. Y. (2001). *What are the risk factors and protective factors considered by approved social workers in determining the compulsory admission of patients in psychiatric emergencies in Hong Kong?* Master of Social Science Dissertation, Department of Social Work and Social Administration, The University of Hong Kong.

Lawson, J. S. (1995). Hong Kong mental health services—A review—1994. *Hong Kong Journal of Mental Health, 24,* 14-24.

Leff, J. Kuipers, L., Berkowitz, R., Eberlein-Vries, R., & Sturgeon, D. (1982). A controlled trial of social intervention in the families of schizophrenic patients. *British Journal of Psychiatry, 141,* 121-134.

Leff, J. P. & Vaughn, C. E. (1981). The role of maintenance therapy and relatives' expressed emotion in relapse of schizophrenia: A two-year follow-up. *British Journal of Psychiatry, 139,* 102-104.

Leff, J. P. & Vaughn, C. E. (1985). *Expressed emotion in families.* New York: Guilford Press.

Levine, I. S. & Fleming, M. (1984). *Human resources development: Issues in case management.* Maryland: Human Resource Development.

Liberman, R. P., Neuchterlein, K. H., & Wallace, C. J. (1982). Social skills training and the nature of schizophrenia. In James P. Curran & Peter M. Monti (Eds.), *Social skills training: A practical handbook for assessment and treatment* (pp. 5-57). New York: Guilford Press.

Lindenmayer, J. P., Crowner, M., & Cosgrove, V. (2002). Emergency treatment of agitation and aggression. In M. H. Allen (Ed.), *Review of psychiatry,* Volume 21, *Emergency psychiatry* (pp. 115-150). Washington, DC: American Psychiatric Press.

Livesley, W. J. (Ed.) (2001). *Handbook of personality disorders: Theory, research and treatment.* New York: Guilford Press.

Lukoff, D., Nuechterlein, K. H., & Ventura, J. (1986). Manual for the expanded brief psychiatric rating scale. *Schizophrenia Bulletin, 12,* 594-602.

Marder, S. R. (1986). Depot neuroleptics: Side effects and safety. *Journal of Clinical Psychopharmacology, 6,* 24S-29S.

Maris, R. W. (Ed.) (1992). *Assessment and prediction of suicide.* New York: Guilford Press.

Martin, G. & Pear, J. (1999). *Behavior modification: What it is and how to do it.* Upper Saddle River, NJ: Prentice Hall.

Meichenbaum, D. H. (1986). Cognitive behavior modification. In F. H. Kanfer & A. P. Goldstein (Eds.), *Helping people change: A textbook of methods,* Third edition (pp. 346-380). New York: Pergamon Press.

Merson, S., Tyrer, P., Onyett, S., Lack, S., Birkett, P., Lynch, S., & Johnson, T. (1992). Early intervention in psychiatric emergencies: A controlled clinical trial. *Lancet, 339*(8805), 1311-1314.

Mezzich, J. E. & Zimmer, B. (1990). *Emergency psychiatry.* Madison, CT: International Universities Press.

Moyer, K. E. (1987). *Violence and aggression: A physical perspective.* London: Paragon House.

Mueser, K. T., Bellack, A. S., Morrison, R. L., & Wixted, J. T. (1990). Social competence in schizophrenia: Premorbid adjustment, social skill, and domains of functioning. *Journal of Psychiatric Research, 24,* 51-63.

Mueser, K. T. & Gingerich, S. (1994). *Coping with schizophrenia: A guide for families.* Oakland, CA: New Harbinger Publications, Inc.

National Alliance of the Mentally Ill (NAMI) (2004). About NAMI. Available online at: <http//www.nami.org/template.cfm?section=About_NAMI>.

Nisbet, P. A. (1996). Protective factors for suicidal black females. *Suicide and Life-Threatening Behavior, 26*(4), 325-341.

Noh, S. & Turner, R. J. (1987). Living with psychiatric patients: Implications for mental health of family members. *Social Science Medicine, 25*(3), 71-263.

Pattison, E. M. & Kahan, J. (1983). The deliberate self-harm syndrome. *American Journal of Psychiatry, 140*(7), 867-872.

Pearson, V. (1993). Families in China: An undervalued resource in mental health? *Journal of Family Therapy, 15,* 163-185.

Pearson, V., Nelson, Y., Ip, F., Lo, E., Ho, K. K., & Hui, H. (2003). To tell or not to tell: Disability disclosure and job application outcomes. *The Journal of Rehabilitation, 69*(4), 35-38.

Peurifoy, R. Z. (1995). *Anxiety, phobias and panic: A step-by-step program for regaining control of your life.* New York: Warner Books.

Phillips, M., Xiong, W., & Zhao, Z. (1990). *Issues related to the use of assessment instruments for negative-positive psychiatric symptoms.* Hubei: Science and · Technology Press.

Rapp, C. A. (1998a). The active ingredients of effective case management: A research synthesis. *Community Mental Health Journal, 34*(4), 363-380.

Rapp, C. A. (1998b). *The strengths model: Case management with people suffering from severe and persistent mental illness.* New York: Oxford University Press.

Rogers, C. R. (1961). *On becoming a person: A therapist's view of psychotherapy.* Boston: Houghton Mifflin.

Rogers, C. R. (1980). *A way of being.* Boston: Houghton Mifflin.

Roy, A. (2001). Consumers of mental health services. *Suicide & Life-Threatening Behavior, 31*(Suppl), 60-83.

Santos, A. B., Hawkins, G. D., Julius, B., Deci, P. A., Hiers, T. H., & Burns, B. J. (1993). A pilot study of assertive community treatment for patients with chronic psychotic disorders. *American Journal of Psychiatry, 150*(3), 501-504.

Sarafino, E. P. (2002). *Health psychology.* New York: John Wiley & Sons.

Social Welfare Department (1999). *Operational guidelines on procedures arising from provisions in the Mental Health Ordinance Cap 136.* Hong Kong: Rehabilitation and Medical Social Services Branch.

Spaniol, L., Jung, H., Zipple, A. M., & Fitzgerald, S. (1987). Families as a resource in the rehabilitation of severely psychiatrically disabled. In A. B. Hatfield & H. P. Lefley (Eds.), *Families of the Mentally Ill: Coping and Adaptation.* New York: Guilford Press.

Stefanis, N., Rabe-Hesketh, S., Clark, B., & Bebbington, P. (1999). An evaluation of a psychiatric emergency clinic. *Journal of Mental Health, 8*(1), 29-42.

Sundel, M. & Sundel, S. S. (1998). Psychopharmacological treatment of panic disorder. *Research on Social Work Practice, 8*(4), 426-452.

Taylor, P. J. (1997). Mental disorder and risk of violence. *International Review of Psychiatry, 9,* 2-3, 157-161.

Test, M. A. & Stein, L. I. (2000). Practical guidelines for the community treatment of marked impaired patients. *Community Mental Health Journal, 36*(1), 47-60.

Torrey, E. F. (1988). *Surviving schizophrenia: A family manual.* New York: Harper & Row.

Trower, P., Bryant, B., & Argyle, M. (1986). *Social skills & mental health.* London: Methuen & Co. Ltd.

Tsang, W. H. & Pearson, V. (2001). Work-related social skills training for people with schizophrenia in Hong Kong. *Schizophrenia Bulletin, 27*(1), 139-148.

Tse, J. W. L. (2000). *Youth suicide: Facts, prevention and crisis management.* Hong Kong: The Chinese University of Hong Kong.

Turkat, I. D. (1990). *The personality disorders: A psychological approach to clinical management.* New York: Pergamon Press.

U. S. Public Health Service. (2004). *Mental Health: A Report of the Surgeon General: Medications for Anxiety Disorders.* Available online at: <http://www.surgeongeneral.gov/library/mentalhealth/chapter4/sec2.html>.

Vaccaro, J.V., Pitts, D.B., & Wallace, C.J. (1992). Functional assessment. In R.P. Liberman (Ed.), *Handbook of psychiatric rehabilitation* (pp. 78-94). Boston: Allyn & Bacon.

Walsh, J. (2000). *Clinical case management with persons having mental illness: A relationship-based perspective.* Belmont, CA: Brooks/Cole.

Ward, M. F. (1995). *Nursing the psychiatric emergency.* Boston: Butterworth Heinemann.

Way, B. R. & Banks, S. (2001). Clinical factors related to admission and release decisions in psychiatric emergency services. *Psychiatric Services, 52*(2), 214-218.

Wing, J. K. & Morris, B. (Eds.) (1981). *Handbook of psychiatric rehabilitation practice.* New York: Oxford University Press.

Wong, F. K. D. (2000). Stress factors and mental health of caregivers with relatives suffering from schizophrenia in Hong Kong: Implications for culturally sensitive practices. *British Journal of Social Work, 30,* 365-382.

Wong, F. K. D., Jourbert, L., & Meadows, G. (2002). *A comparative study of burdens, and mental and physical health of careers in Hong Kong and Australia.* Unpublished Manuscript, The University of Hong Kong.

Wong, F. K. D. & Poon, W. L. (2002). Factors influencing expressed emotion found between Chinese caregivers and their relatives with schizophrenia in Hong Kong: A qualitative analysis. *Social Work in Mental Health, 1*(2), 61-81.

Wong, F. K. D., Pui, T. K. H., Pearson, V., and Chiu, S. N. (2003). Changing health beliefs on causations of mental illness and their impacts on family burdens and the mental health of Chinese caregivers in Hong Kong. *International Journal of Mental Health, 32*(2), 84-98.

World Health Organization (1992). *The ICD-10 classification of mental and behavioural disorders: Clinical descriptions and diagnostic guidelines.* Geneva: World Health Organization.

Yalom, I. D. (1980). *Existential psychotherapy.* New York: Basic Books.

Yank, G. R., Bentley, K. J., and Hargrove, D. S. (1993). The vulnerability-stress model of schizophrenia: Advances in psychosocial treatment. *American Journal of Orthpsychiatry, 63*(1), 55-69.

Yip, K. S. (1997). An overview of the development of psychiatric rehabilitation services in Hong Kong. *Hong Kong Journal of Mental Health, 26,* 8-27.

Yip, K. S. (1998). A historical review of mental health services in Hong Kong (1841-1995). *International Journal of Social Psychiatry, 44*(1), 46-55.

Yip, P. S. F. & Tan, R. C. E. (1998). Suicides in Hong-Kong and Singapore: A tale of two cities. *International Journal of Social Psychiatry, 44*(4), 267-279.

Young, M. A., Fogg, L. F., Scheftner, W., Fawcett, J., Akiskal, H., & Maser, J. (1996). Stable trait components of hopelessness: Baseline and sensitivity to depression. *Journal of Abnormal Psychology, 105*(2), 155-165.

Zhang, M., He, Y. L., Gittleman, M., Wong, Z., & Yan, H. Q. (1998). Group psychoeducation of relatives of schizophrenic patients: Two-year experiences. *Psychiatry and Clinical Neurosciences, 52,* 344-347.

Index

Page numbers followed by the letter "f" indicate figures; those followed by the letter "t" indicate tables.